Table of Contents

Argyll Clinic: A Medical Office Simulation is designed to provide the student with practical exposure to activities that might be encountered on the job in a medical office environment. In addition, the activities contained in this simulation will reinforce many of the topics covered in a medical office procedures subject.

By following individual project instructions and using the Argyll Clinic Procedures Manual provided, students should be able to successfully complete all the assignments within a specified time frame. Many of the tasks in the projects are intended for use with different computer applications: these include word processing and electronic appointment scheduling.

Forms that are required for this simulation are enclosed, and an Argyll letterhead template and medical transcription files are available on the CD accompanying this package.

Argyll Clinic: A Medical Office Simulation

Agnes Seaton
Seneca College of Applied Arts and Technology, Toronto

Nancy Elder
Seneca College of Applied Arts and Technology, Toronto

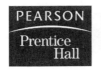

PEARSON
Prentice Hall

PRENTICE HALL HEALTH

Toronto

National Library of Canada Cataloguing in Publication

Seaton, Agnes
    Argyll Clinic : a medical office simulation / Agnes Seaton, Nancy Elder. -- 1st ed.

ISBN 0-13-177092-6

    1. Medical offices--Management--Problems, exercises, etc. 2. Medical secretaries--
Problems, exercises, etc. I. Elder, Nancy II. Title.

R728.8.S42 2005   651'.961   C2004-901845-0

ISBN 0-13-177092-6

Vice President, Editorial Director: Michael J. Young
Executive Acquisitions Editor: Samantha Scully
Marketing Manager: Cas Shields
Senior Developmental Editor: Paul Donnelly
Production Editor: Judith Scott
Production Coordinator: Deborah Starks
Page Layout: Agnes Seaton and Nancy Elder
Art Director: Mary Opper
Interior and Cover Design: Anthony Leung
Cover Image: PhotoDisc

13   16

Printed and bound in Canada

Acknowledgements

We are extremely grateful for all the help we received when we ventured into the unknown realm of authorship. In particular, there are a few people we would like to acknowledge for the help so generously extended to us.

First and foremost, special thanks must go to Dr. Chris Gannage and Dr. Norma Yoneyama whose contributions were key to getting us started on the simulation in the first place.

We owe a debt of gratitude to Liz Watt and Valerie Thompson, who both said that this simulation was a worthwhile project and were brave enough to put their words into action by using Argyll Clinic as a teaching tool. Our sincere appreciation to Kent Peel for his "vocal" contribution!

Also, thanks to Karin Barnett of *Medcom Solutions,* who generously shared information with us.

Thanks to Samantha Scully, who was interested in our simulation from the first glimpse of it and who encouraged us when we were floundering and felt like giving up. To Paul Donnelly, our trusty editor, who did not seem to mind the use of Scottish names in spite of his Irish heritage, thanks for all the help. To Deborah Starks, who had to explain to us frequently the intricacies of the printing process, thank you for your assistance. To Judith Scott, many thanks; your unruffled composure helped calm down two anxious authors.

To Bob—thanks for climbing Kilimanjaro to take the photograph for the cheques! To Jim—thanks for the maps to ensure we did not get lost on our "educational trips"! To John McCulloch—thanks for coming to our rescue after Bob's camera broke!

We said on many occasions that if we had known how much work was involved in this project, we would never have started it in the first place. However, all that work will have been worth it if we have helped, in some measure, to prepare medical office administration students to experience the reality of working successfully in a medical office.

A and N

Argyll Clinic

OVERVIEW

PROJECT OVERVIEW

Argyll Clinic: A Medical Office Simulation consists of a series of projects that covers a period of five days in a medical office. It is estimated that these projects will require approximately 20-25 hours to complete, depending upon the ability of the student. To maximize the benefits of this package, it is recommended that the simulation be used in its project-based format, as some of the activities are ongoing over several days. However, it should be noted that it is possible to use some of the activities as stand-alone tasks.

All information and materials required to complete the project assignments are contained in this workbook or on the accompanying CD. A total of six file folders and labels are provided for student use.

The two file folders (with end tabs) and the colored folder inserts are to be used for patient charts in Project 3. Alpha labels, file folder labels, and index tabs are also provided for this project.

Four file folders and file folder labels are provided for organization of student work and should be labeled as follows:

- Current Assignments
- Completed Assignments   (to be submitted for evaluation)
- Evaluated Projects 1-5   (to file completed and graded material)
- Reference Materials   (to store calendar, abbreviations, etc.)

The goal of this simulation is to provide on-the-job training and experience for students who are planning a career as a medical administrative assistant or a medical secretary. This simulation provides a realistic medical office setting for students as the activities have been selected from offices of primary care practitioners.

By creating this realistic environment, students gain practical experience by performing a variety of tasks designed to develop sound decision-making skills and critical thinking skills. These tasks incorporate the theory taught in a medical office procedures subject.

It is recommended that students work independently on tasks under instructor-controlled conditions in order to effectively simulate an actual office setting.

PROJECTS

- Each project represents one day's activities in the clinic.

- By following individual project instructions and by using the Argyll Clinic Procedures Manual provided, students should be able to successfully complete all the assignments within a specified time frame. Many of the tasks in the projects are intended for use with different computer applications: these include word processing and electronic appointment scheduling.

EVALUATION

- Each of the five projects is accompanied by a detailed instruction sheet that is also designed to be used by the instructor for evaluation purposes.

PROCEDURES MANUAL

- This section establishes the scenario for the Argyll Clinic and gives the pertinent data about the primary care practitioners, the associate physicians, and office personnel.

- It also outlines information on the procedures to be adhered to in the office.

- In addition, it contains a detailed job description outlining duties and responsibilities of clerical staff.

- Reference sources that are needed to complete some of the tasks are included in the manual. These include items such as payroll guidelines, a six-month calendar, and appointment scheduling guidelines.

Argyll Clinic

PROCEDURES MANUAL

INTRODUCTION

Congratulations! You are employed as the Medical Administrative Assistant in the Argyll Clinic, which provides medical services in a suburban community in the northeast part of Toronto.

Our mission is to provide optimum health care to the individuals and families whom we see, in a responsible, effective, and caring manner; therefore, our interaction with our clientele should reflect this philosophy. Remember, the first impression given to patients by our medical staff sets the overall tone of the practice.

Staff should work together in a cooperative manner. Staff members may have their areas of expertise (i.e., billing, clinical); however, there should be enough sharing of information to enable staff to "pinch hit" for one another during illnesses, holidays, and during peak office periods. The overall goal, as stated above, is to provide a responsible, effective, and caring medical environment for our clients.

CLINIC INFORMATION

In the clinic the following three primary care practitioners provide family medical services to their patients:

- Craig Cameron, MD, CCFP
- Bruce G. Findlay, MD, FRCPC
- Lewis A. Durant, MD

The following is a listing of the personnel who make up the office staff:

- Maureen Jones, RN
- Your Professor, who is the Office Manager
- Your Name, Medical Administrative Assistant
- Julie Tassopoulos, CMS, Medical Office Assistant (Part-Time)

ASSOCIATE PHYSICIANS

In addition, there are associate physicians who use the administrative services of the clinic, and you are responsible for providing them with administrative assistance (e.g., transcribing consultation letters and patient reports) when necessary. The following is a list of these practitioners:

Arlene Baird, MD, FACS, FRCSC	Shirley A. Chung, MD, MRCP, FRCPC
Margaret Baird, MD, FRCOG, FRCS, FRCSC	Brinder Rahman, MD, FRCSC
Jane C. Bennett, MD, FRCPC	Catharine Russell, MD, FACP, FRCPC
James S. Driuna, MD, FACS, FRCSC	Alice Turner, MD

APPOINTMENT SCHEDULING GUIDELINES

Appointments are 15 minutes per patient except for the following, which require a half-hour appointment:

- Complete physical exam (CPX)
- Annual health exam (AHE)
- New patients
- Counselling
- Chest pain
- First obstetrical visit

NOTE:

- Injections should be fitted in between appointments

- Allow a time slot for Coffee/Messages in the morning and in the afternoon

- If the doctor is in the office for a full day (i.e., from 9 or 10 a.m. to 5. p.m.), then block off a one-hour lunch break from 12 noon to 1 p.m.

- Please note that Dr. Findlay is the resident family practitioner for Strone Nursing Home. He routinely visits the residents on Wednesday afternoons.

- You should prepare a Day Sheet for each doctor, showing the scheduled appointments for the next day, before you leave the office. A sample Day Sheet is provided for your information.

PAYROLL GUIDELINES

- In the Argyll Clinic, as is standard procedure in many physicians' offices, payroll is processed manually.

- As part of the payroll process, you must maintain an Employee Payroll Record for each individual member of staff.

- Staff at the Argyll Clinic is paid on an hourly basis; therefore, to calculate the gross wage, multiply the number of hours worked in the pay period by the hourly rate.

- Daily hours of work must be recorded on the Employee Payroll Record.

- Pay periods at the clinic are bi-weekly (26 pay periods per annum) with cheques being issued every second Friday.

- Source deductions tables (CPP, EI, and income tax) are included for use with the payroll assignment.

- An Employee Payroll Statement must, by law, be prepared for each employee for each pay period.

PROOFREADERS' MARKS

Proofreading Mark	Usage	Revision
] [Centre	] Argyll Clinic [	Argyll Clinic
] Move right	]Argyll Clinic	Argyll Clinic
[Move left	[Argyll Clinic	Argyll Clinic
¶ New paragraph	. . .hospital for tests. ¶ Surgery is scheduled. . .	. . .hospital for tests. Surgery is scheduled. . .
# Insert space ^	# Historyand Physical ^	History and Physical
^ Insert word	and History Physical ^	History and Physical
◯ Spell out in full	(Exam)	Examination
lc / Lowercase	lc Complete the Report. . .	Complete the report. . .
uc ＿ Uppercase	uc argyll Clinic	Argyll Clinic
. . . . . Stet—do not delete	I am ~~really~~ delighted. . . Stet	I am really delighted. . .
ù Insert a period	this patientù Please. . .	. . . this patient. Please. . .
⟲ Transpose	It is only the . . .	It is the only. . .
⌣ Close up	path ⌣ ology	pathology
(ital) ＿＿＿ Italics	(ital) OMSA-HCA Communiqué	*Communiqué*
(bold) 〰〰 Bold	(bold) Argyll Clinic 〰〰〰	**Argyll Clinic**

POSTAL ABBREVIATIONS
FOR PROVINCES AND TERRITORIES

Province	Abbreviation
Alberta	AB
British Columbia	BC
Manitoba	MB
New Brunswick	NB
Newfoundland and Labrador	NF
Northwest Territories	NT
Nova Scotia	NS
Nunavut	NU
Ontario	ON
Prince Edward Island	PE
Quebec	QC
Saskatchewan	SK
Yukon	YT

ABBREVIATIONS FOR ARGYLL CLINIC

Abbreviation	Meaning	Abbreviation	Meaning
AC	Argyll Clinic	MCHC	Mean corpuscular hemoglobin concentration
AHE	Annual health examination	MCV	Mean corpuscular volume
b.i.d.	Twice a day	MOHLTC	Ministry of Health and Long-term Care
Chol	Cholesterol	MOT	Ministry of Transport
CMS	Certified Medical Secretary	MSK	Musculoskeletal system
CPX	Complete physical examination	MVA	Motor Vehicle Accident
CPP	Canada Pension Plan	OA	Osteoarthritis
CVS	Cardiovascular system	OMA	Ontario Medical Association
EI	**Employment Insurance**	OMSA—HCA	**Ontario Medical Secretaries Association—Health Care Associates**
FBS	Fasting blood sugar	PA	Posteroanterior
HDL	High-density lipoprotein	RBC	Red blood cell (count)
LDL	Low-density lipoprotein	RIA	Radioimmunoassay
LMP	Last menstrual period	TSH	Thyroid-stimulating hormone
MCH	Mean corpuscular hemoglobin	WBC	White blood cell (count)

DUTIES AND RESPONSIBILITIES OF MEDICAL STAFF

It is of prime importance that office staff ensures the Argyll Clinic runs smoothly, that patients are treated in an effective and caring manner, and that doctors' times are optimally utilized.

RECEPTION AND CLERICAL DUTIES

- Receive and/or register patients and obtain pertinent data politely, quickly, and efficiently
- Register patients and prepare charts
- Screen incoming telephone calls and take messages
- Book appointments appropriately
- Phone recalls and follow-up appointments
- Telephone pharmacies with doctor-approved prescription reorders
- Book appointments for referrals to specialists, notify patients of specialist appointments, and make appropriate notations on patient charts
- Book investigative procedures and tests at diagnostic imaging clinics (i.e., CT scan, x-ray, ultrasound)
- Arrange time for pharmaceutical representatives to consult with doctors
- Make certain that the reception area is neat and tidy
- Record after hours voice message; retrieve and respond to incoming messages in a prompt manner
- Stock office supplies as required (i.e., stationery, appointment cards)
- Photocopy documents as needed
- Prepare patient charts using colour-coded labels and stickers
- File charts in alphabetical order
- File lab results, medical correspondence, and x-ray results behind appropriate folder inserts, ensuring that small loose sheets are attached to an 8.5" by 11" sheet of paper.
- Transcribe all required patient reports and correspondence (i.e., medical/legal reports, chart notes, etc.)
- Prepare day sheets; continually update as required
- Pull charts for next day and date stamp Clinical Data Sheets
- Photocopy charts of patients who are transferring to another medical facility

BILLING

- Perform billing tasks on a daily basis (MOHLTC and non-insured services)
- Send in submissions weekly
- Perform monthly reconciliation tasks
- Establish liaison with Ministry of Health and Long-Term Care

CLINICAL

- Ensure examination rooms are prepared and ready for use; check rooms between patient appointments
- Direct patients to examination rooms
- Ensure that examining rooms are adequately stocked
- Organize and store drug samples
- Sterilize equipment in the autoclave located in the nursing station
- Ensure educational material is available for patients
- Assist with prenatal visits (i.e., fill in forms, record weight, and test urine for glucose)
- Assist with physical examinations (i.e., record weight, height, etc.)
- Retrieve immunization cards for update
- Perform visual acuity testing when needed
- Ensure swabs are properly labeled and lab requisition forms are correctly completed

BOOKKEEPING

- Record all sundry expenses in the Petty Cash Book, balance the Petty Cash on a monthly basis, and replenish the fund
- Record transactions in the Cash Disbursements Journal and prepare signature. Balance the Cash Disbursements on a monthly basis.
- Prepare bi-weekly payroll and cheques for employees
- Ensure that all receipts are stored and books are up to date for year-end tax preparation

CALENDAR

July	Sun	Mon	Tue	Wed	Thu	Fri	Sat
							1
	2	3	4	5	6	7	8
	9	10	11	12	13	14	15
	16	17	18	19	20	21	22
	23	24	25	26	27	28	29
	30	31					

August	Sun	Mon	Tue	Wed	Thu	Fri	Sat
			1	2	3	4	5
	6	7	8	9	10	11	12
	13	14	15	16	17	18	19
	20	21	22	23	24	25	26
	27	28	29	30	31		

September	Sun	Mon	Tue	Wed	Thu	Fri	Sat
						1	2
	3	4	5	6	7	8	9
	10	11	12	13	14	15	16
	17	18	19	20	21	22	23
	24	25	26	27	28	29	30

October	Sun	Mon	Tue	Wed	Thu	Fri	Sat
	1	2	3	4	5	6	7
	8	9	10	11	12	13	14
	15	16	17	18	19	20	21
	22	23	24	25	26	27	28
	29	30	31				

November	Sun	Mon	Tue	Wed	Thu	Fri	Sat
				1	2	3	4
	5	6	7	8	9	10	11
	12	13	14	15	16	17	18
	19	20	21	22	23	24	25
	26	27	28	29	30		

December	Sun	Mon	Tue	Wed	Thu	Fri	Sat
						1	2
	3	4	5	6	7	8	9
	10	11	12	13	14	15	16
	17	18	19	20	21	22	23
	24	25	26	27	28	29	30
	31						

PATIENT DATABASE INFORMATION

1. ALEXANDER, WILLIAM R.

770 Cowal Place
TORONTO, ON   F4T 5N6

SEX:	MALE
DOB:	03/07/1977
MOH NO.:	4562 873 069
HOME:	555-2734
BUSINESS:	555-4842

5. BOYD, EWAN

245 Auchamore Road
TORONTO, ON   F2T 1N3

SEX:	MALE
DOB:	22/01/1979
MOH NO.:	2134 418 918
HOME:	555-1308
BUSINESS:	555-3807

2. ARMSTRONG, SANDRA M.

6 Royal Crescent
TORONTO, ON   F9T 9N3

SEX:	FEMALE
DOB:	13/01/1982
MOH NO.:	9930 614 392
HOME:	555-9644
BUSINESS:	555-2591

6. BURNS, JULIE L.

588 Kirn Boulevard
TORONTO, ON   F6T 8N4

SEX:	FEMALE
DOB:	22/02/1972
MOH NO.:	6553 614 691
HOME:	555-2888
BUSINESS:	555-2675

3. BEATTIE, ROBERT GLEN

1010 Dumbarton Road
TORONTO, ON   F8T 9N5

SEX:	MALE
DOB:	11/11/1992
MOH NO.:	8955 119 832 LL
HOME:	555-9547

7. BURNS, MARSHALL D.

588 Kirn Boulevard
TORONTO, ON   F6T 8N4

SEX:	MALE
DOB:	30/10/1981
MOH NO.:	6848 348 972
HOME:	555-2888
BUSINESS:	555-6408

4. BLAIR, COLIN J.

5 Montrose Avenue
TORONTO, ON   F3T 7N1

SEX:	MALE
DOB:	15/08/1969
MOH NO.:	3714 136 078
HOME:	555-0139
BUSINESS:	555-5131

8. CAIRNS, RHONA

90 Logan Street North
TORONTO, ON   F1T 8N8

SEX:	FEMALE
DOB:	06/10/1978
MOH NO.:	1881 341 232
HOME:	555-8174
BUSINESS:	555-2462

9.	**CAMERON, JACQUELINE**		13.	**HAMILTON, SKYE J.**

9.   CAMERON, JACQUELINE

17 Argyll Street
TORONTO, ON   F2T 1N8

SEX:	FEMALE
DOB:	16/05/1978
MOH No.:	2158 029 435
HOME:	555-2776
BUSINESS:	555-8049

13.   HAMILTON, SKYE J.

5A Marine Parade
TORONTO, ON   F9T 9N5

SEX:	FEMALE
DOB:	24/10/1978
MOH No.:	9959 048 670
HOME:	555-5065
BUSINESS:	555-3906

10.   COLANGELO, ANITA

463 Vistaview Road
TORONTO, ON   F6Z 3L5

SEX:	FEMALE
DOB:	14/01/1945
MOH No.:	7777 777 777
HOME:	555-1314
BUSINESS:	555-1632

14.   HARRIS, KATRINA C.

494 Highland Avenue
TORONTO, ON   F2T 1N7

SEX:	FEMALE
DOB:	27/08/1976
MOH No.:	2177 974 371
HOME:	555-0227
BUSINESS:	555-7683

11.   DUNCAN, ELISE S.

628 Hunter's Quay
TORONTO, ON   F6T 2N3

SEX:	FEMALE
DOB:	19/04/1998
MOH No.:	6293 685 050 XY
HOME:	555-9359
BUSINESS:	555-4008

15.   KERR, FIONA L.

82 Ferry Brae
TORONTO, ON   F2T 0N8

SEX:	FEMALE
DOB:	17/03/1965
MOH No.:	2083 365 532
HOME:	555-6940
BUSINESS:	555-3780

12.   FRASER, MORAG

101 Moir Street
TORONTO, ON   F4T 2N2

SEX:	FEMALE
DOB:	04/12/1999
MOH No.:	4229 132 974
HOME:	555-4418

16.   KLEIN, BRANDY

One Hillfoot Street
TORONTO, ON   F2T 8N5

SEX:	FEMALE
DOB:	21/08/1978
MOH No.:	2853 708 317 DG
HOME:	555-4746
BUSINESS:	555-8945

Procedures Manual

17.	LEWIS, JEAN

6073 Ardenslate Road
TORONTO, ON   F6T 2N5

SEX: FEMALE
DOB: 01/04/1980
MOH NO.:   6253 567 918

HOME: 555-0791
BUSINESS: 555-3254

18. MACKENZIE, LISA J.

35 Hamilton Street
TORONTO, ON   F4T 8N3

SEX: FEMALE
DOB: 07/11/1973
MOH NO.:   4830 540 177

HOME: 555-0393
BUSINESS: 555-3316

19. MCBETH, GAVIN

21 Kirk Street
TORONTO, ON   F7T 2N1

SEX: MALE
DOB: 02/02/1981
MOH NO.:   7211 265 132

HOME: 555-3886
BUSINESS: 555-3518

20. MUIR, ROSS A.

2516 Sandbank Road
TORONTO, ON   F1T 9N9

SEX: MALE
DOB: 12/11/1974
MOH NO.:   1991 024 892

HOME: 555-7683
BUSINESS: 555-6741

21. NICHOLSON, CLAIRE K.

7 Clyde Street
TORONTO, ON   F1T 6N4

SEX: FEMALE
DOB: 11/03/1977
MOH NO.:   1643 304 957

HOME: 555-8069
BUSINESS: 555-5050

22. ROBERTS, KENNETH M.

7 Milton Estate Road
TORONTO, ON   F9T 9N9

SEX: MALE
DOB: 26/03/1982
MOH NO.:   9997 829 735

HOME: 555-1481
BUSINESS: 555-4579

23. ROBINSON, SCOTT

36 Castle Gardens Road
TORONTO, ON   F5T 1N0

SEX: MALE
DOB: 26/05/1950
MOH NO.:   5101 830 452

HOME: 555-2183
BUSINESS: 555-2942

24. SCOTT, IAIN J.

92 Simpson Avenue
TORONTO, ON   F8T 0N4

SEX: MALE
DOB: 21/11/1985
MOH NO.:   8082 435 291

HOME: 555-1748
BUSINESS: 555-6921

25.	SHEARLAW, CRAIG ROBERT	29.	VON SCHROEDER, HANS

25. SHEARLAW, CRAIG ROBERT

22 Kirkland Street
TORONTO, ON   F7T 4N2

SEX:	MALE
DOB:	07/01/1992
MOH No.:	7427 993 717

| HOME: | 555-9733 |

29. VON SCHROEDER, HANS

351 Longmore Street
TORONTO, ON   F2X 2J5

Sex:	Male
DOB:	01/01/1940
MOH No.:	9999 999 999

| Home: | 555-9429 |
| BUSINESS: | 555-1210 |

26. SUTHERLAND, DEIRDRE

45 McArthur Street
TORONTO, ON   F4T 4N4

SEX:	FEMALE
DOB:	15/12/1930
MOH No.:	4429 869 557

| HOME: | 555-4580 |

30. WILSON, Lindsay

76B East Kilbride Avenue
TORONTO, ON   F3T 5N5

SEX:	FEMALE
DOB:	08/04/1972
MOH No.:	3559 892 397

| HOME: | 555-9642 |
| BUSINESS: | 555-0261 |

27. URQUHART, BARBARA J.

71 Victoria Parade
TORONTO, ON   F4T 9N0

SEX:	FEMALE
DOB:	09/06/1975
MOH No.:	4908 006 333

| HOME: | 555-5764 |
| BUSINESS: | 555-7408 |

31 ZABISEWSKI, MEREDITH

87A Midge Lane
TORONTO, ON   F6Q 9S4

SEX:	FEMALE
DOB:	13/10/2000
MOH No.:	1393 486 095 AB

| HOME: | 555-6522 |

28. VANBERKEL, MICHAEL

85 Gantocks Road
TORONTO, ON   F7T 9N7

SEX:	MALE
DOB:	14/10/1968
MOH No.:	7979 791 279

| HOME: | 555-2621 |
| BUSINESS: | 555-1698 |

32 ZABISEWSKI, PAIGE

87A Midge Lane
TORONTO, ON   F6Q 9S4

SEX:	FEMALE
DOB:	13/10/2000
MOH No.:	4444 444 444 DC

| HOME: | 555-6522 |

Argyll Clinic

PROJECT 1

Instruction/Evaluation Sheet

NAME _____   DATE _____

TASK	INSTRUCTIONS - PROJECT 1	FOR STUDENT'S USE		FOR INSTRUCTOR'S USE	
		YES	NO	ERRORS	TOTAL
1	Copy Argyll Letterhead template from Argyll Disk to your student disk.				
2	Using this template, correctly update the **Clinic Information** that is located in Project 1. There are several handwritten changes on the document that must be accommodated in the final copy. In addition, the following instructions **must** be followed when completing this assignment:				
	• Use 12-point Times New Roman font for the body, and use any sans serif font for the headings.				
	• If the finished document exceeds one page, keyboard an appropriate second-page header.				
	• Use an appropriate and consistent document format.				
	• Ensure document is free of keyboarding errors.				
	• Ensure appropriate document name is indicated in reference line in a footer and print one copy.				
3	Set up the appointment book for the week of August 28-September 1. Use the Appointment Scheduling Guidelines (contained in the Procedures Manual) and the office hours (included in the updated Argyll Information Sheet) for this task.				

		FOR STUDENT'S USE		FOR INSTRUCTOR'S USE	
TASK	**INSTRUCTIONS - PROJECT 1**	**YES**	**NO**	**ERRORS**	**TOTAL**
	INCOMING APPOINTMENT REQUESTS				
4	On the appointment schedule, block off the times (as indicated below) the doctors will be out of the clinic.				
	• Dr. Findlay will be out of the office all day on Friday as he is attending a conference organized by the OMA at the Park Plaza Hotel.				
	• Dr. Cameron is a guest speaker at the monthly dinner meeting of the local chapter of the OMSA – HCA. The meeting is scheduled for 5:30 p.m. on Wednesday. His last appointment of the day should be at 4 p.m.				
5	Book appointments for the following patients with the doctor specified.				
	• Gavin McBeth has a wart on his left foot (555-3886) and wants an appointment with Dr. Cameron on Wednesday after 3 p.m.				
	• Katrina Harris (555-0227) requests first obstetrical visit with Dr. Findlay on Tuesday afternoon.				
	• Colin Blair has persistent diarrhea (555-0139) and requests a Monday afternoon appointment with Dr. Findlay				
	• Lisa MacKenzie (555-0393), requesting CPX appointment on Wednesday with Dr. Findlay.				
	• Fiona Kerr (555-6940) constipation x3 days asks for Monday morning appointment with Dr. Cameron.				

Instruction/Evaluation Sheet

TASK	INSTRUCTIONS - PROJECT 1	FOR STUDENT'S USE		FOR INSTRUCTOR'S USE	
		YES	NO	ERRORS	TOTAL
	INCOMING APPOINTMENT REQUESTS				
	• Rhona Cairns (555-8174) painful cystitis, would like Monday a.m., Dr. Findlay				
	• Iain Scott, sore left knee, (555-1748). Requesting appointment late in the day on Friday with Dr. Cameron.				
	• Julie Burns and Marshall Burns (555-2888), both patients of Dr. Cameron would like a Friday appointment for allergy shots				
	• Scott Robinson wants to talk to Dr. Cameron. He is upset about his son's drinking problem (555-2942). He prefers Monday afternoon appointment, if possible.				
	• Sandra Armstrong has recurring pain in right shoulder (555-2591) requesting Tuesday appointment with Dr. Cameron				
	• Barbara Urquhart, severe earache, Monday a.m. appointment, Dr. Findlay (555-7408).				
	• Hans Von Schroeder needs a BP check on Friday afternoon after 3 p.m. with Dr. Cameron (555-9429).				

FOR PROFESSOR'S USE ONLY

ARGYLL CLINIC

2999 RENFIELD STREET
TORONTO, ON F2L 4X6

TELEPHONE: (416) 555-2334
FAX: (416) 555-2445

CLINIC INFORMATION

OFFICE HOURS

Note headings in the body of doc. all caps, bold, and centred

For appointment scheduling purposes, the hours of the clinic are as follows:

Doctor	Monday	Tuesday	Wednesday	Thursday	Friday
Findlay	9:00-5:00	9:00-5:00	9:00-1:00	9:00-5:00	9:00-1:00

DAY	DR. CAMERON
Monday	10 to 5 p.m.
Tuesday	10 a.m. to –1 p.m.
Wed	1:00-5:00
Thurs	10 to 5 p.m.
Friday	10 to 5 p.m.

DR. DURRANT

Mon	9:00-5:00
Tues	9:00-1:00
Wednesday	9-5:00
Thurs	9:00-1:00
Friday	10:00-2 p.m.

use table set up please

AFTER HOURS

When our office is closed, you may leave a message on our voice mail, and we will return your call as soon as possible. If you have an urgent problem that cannot wait until the next day, you may go directly to the Kilmun Regional Health Centre. *bold and underline*

APPOINTMENTS

We make every effort to be on time for your appointment. You can help us stay on schedule by:

number the items

- Not dropping in to the office and expecting to be seen.
- Briefly informing the secretary of the reason for your visit, e.g., complete physical, talk, sore throat, headache, and prescription renewal.
- If more than one family member is to be seen kindly telling us beforehand
- Arriving for your appointment on time.

TELEPHONE CALLS

We request that you do not expect advice from your doctor over the telephone. It is difficult, if not impossible, to accurately diagnose and treat you by telephone. Telephone advice is discouraged by the Canadian Medical Protective Association and not recognized by our Provincial Health Care Plan (OHIP) as a service to patients.

PRESCRIPTIONS

bold and underline

It is the new policy that the doctors will not routinely reorder prescription medication over the telephone. If you feel that you require a refill of a prescription medication, please give the office at least a few days' notice so that an appointment can be made for you. If a telephone prescription refill is deemed appropriate, please be advised that this service is not covered by OHIP, and there will be a charge for this uninsured service.

Laboratory And Test Results

bold and italics

We do not phone you with normal results. Our policy is "No news is good news." If a test is abnormal, you will be contacted. However, if you wish to follow-up your results, you are free to phone us or make an appointment.

UNINSURED SERVICES

Certain services that we provide are not included under OHIP. A list of uninsured services is displayed at the reception area. You will be informed when a charge is to be made.

Outside commitments

in full

All three doctors are on Active Staff at Kilmun (Reg.) Health Centre. The staff appointment requires a number of commitments including attendance at weekly educational conferences and administrative meetings.

APPOINTMENT BOOK

Argyll Clinic

Dr. Craig Cameron
Dr. Bruce Findlay

AG

DR CAMERON DATE: _____

TIME	PATIENT
9:00	
9:15	
9:30	
9:45	
10:00	
10:15	
10:30	
10:45	
11:00	
11:15	
11:30	
11:45	
12:00	
12:15	
12:30	
12:45	

REMARKS

AG

TIME	PATIENT
1:00	
1:15	
1:30	
1:45	
2:00	
2:15	
2:30	
2:45	
3:00	
3:15	
3:30	
3:45	
4:00	
4:15	
4:30	
4:45	

REMARKS

AC

Dr Findlay   **Date:** _____   **AC**

TIME	PATIENT	TIME	PATIENT
9:00			
9:15			
9:30			
9:45			
10:00		1:00	
10:15		1:15	
10:30		1:30	
10:45		1:45	
11:00		2:00	
11:15		2:15	
11:30		2:30	
11:45		2:45	
12:00		3:00	
12:15		3:15	
12:30		3:30	
12:45		3:45	
		4:00	
		4:15	
		4:30	
		4:45	
REMARKS		**REMARKS**	

AC **AC**

Dr Cameron   **Date:** _____

Time	Patient	Time	Patient
9:00		1:00	
9:15		1:15	
9:30		1:30	
9:45		1:45	
10:00		2:00	
10:15		2:15	
10:30		2:30	
10:45		2:45	
11:00		3:00	
11:15		3:15	
11:30		3:30	
11:45		3:45	
12:00		4:00	
12:15		4:15	
12:30		4:30	
12:45		4:45	

Remarks

Remarks

AC   Dr Findlay   Date:_____   **AC**

TIME	PATIENT		TIME	PATIENT
9:00			1:00	
9:15			1:15	
9:30			1:30	
9:45			1:45	
10:00			2:00	
10:15			2:15	
10:30			2:30	
10:45			2:45	
11:00			3:00	
11:15			3:15	
11:30			3:30	
11:45			3:45	
12:00			4:00	
12:15			4:15	
12:30			4:30	
12:45			4:45	
REMARKS			REMARKS	

Dr Cameron   Date: _____

Time	Patient
9:00	
9:15	
9:30	
9:45	
10:00	
10:15	
10:30	
10:45	
11:00	
11:15	
11:30	
11:45	
12:00	
12:15	
12:30	
12:45	

REMARKS

Time	Patient
1:00	
1:15	
1:30	
1:45	
2:00	
2:15	
2:30	
2:45	
3:00	
3:15	
3:30	
3:45	
4:00	
4:15	
4:30	
4:45	

REMARKS

AC   DR FINDLAY   DATE:_____   **AC**

TIME	PATIENT	REMARKS	TIME	PATIENT	REMARKS
9:00			1:00		
9:15			1:15		
9:30			1:30		
9:45			1:45		
10:00			2:00		
10:15			2:15		
10:30			2:30		
10:45			2:45		
11:00			3:00		
11:15			3:15		
11:30			3:30		
11:45			3:45		
12:00			4:00		
12:15			4:15		
12:30			4:30		
12:45			4:45		

AC

DR CAMERON   DATE: _____

AC

TIME	PATIENT
9:00	
9:15	
9:30	
9:45	
10:00	
10:15	
10:30	
10:45	
11:00	
11:15	
11:30	
11:45	
12:00	
12:15	
12:30	
12:45	

REMARKS

TIME	PATIENT
1:00	
1:15	
1:30	
1:45	
2:00	
2:15	
2:30	
2:45	
3:00	
3:15	
3:30	
3:45	
4:00	
4:15	
4:30	
4:45	

REMARKS

AC

Dr Findlay   Date: _____

TIME	PATIENT		TIME	PATIENT	
9:00			1:00		
9:15			1:15		
9:30			1:30		
9:45			1:45		
10:00			2:00		
10:15			2:15		
10:30			2:30		
10:45			2:45		
11:00			3:00		
11:15			3:15		
11:30			3:30		
11:45			3:45		
12:00			4:00		
12:15			4:15		
12:30			4:30		
12:45			4:45		
REMARKS			REMARKS		

AC

Dr Cameron   Date: _____

Time	Patient		Time	Patient
9:00			1:00	
9:15			1:15	
9:30			1:30	
9:45			1:45	
10:00			2:00	
10:15			2:15	
10:30			2:30	
10:45			2:45	
11:00			3:00	
11:15			3:15	
11:30			3:30	
11:45			3:45	
12:00			4:00	
12:15			4:15	
12:30			4:30	
12:45			4:45	
Remarks			Remarks	

AC Dr Findlay   Date: _____

TIME	PATIENT	TIME	PATIENT
9:00		1:00	
9:15		1:15	
9:30		1:30	
9:45		1:45	
10:00		2:00	
10:15		2:15	
10:30		2:30	
10:45		2:45	
11:00		3:00	
11:15		3:15	
11:30		3:30	
11:45		3:45	
12:00		4:00	
12:15		4:15	
12:30		4:30	
12:45		4:45	
REMARKS		REMARKS	

Argyll Clinic

PROJECT 2

NAME _____ **DATE** _____

TASK	INSTRUCTIONS - PROJECT 2	FOR STUDENT'S USE		FOR INSTRUCTORS USE	
		YES	NO	ERRORS	TOTAL
1	Prepare a notice showing the office-hours (refer to Project 1 Clinic Information) that will be posted on the patient information notice board in the reception area. This should be set up attractively for readability.				
2	Using the Argyll Letterhead template, prepare the Uninsured Services notice contained in Project 2. As this will be posted on a notice board, it should be a one-page document that is set up appropriately for readability.				
3	Book appointments for the following patients with the doctor specified.				
	• Jacqueline Cameron needs an appointment on Wednesday morning regarding vaginitis (555-2776) – Dr. Findlay.				
	• Anita Colangelo requests a late appointment on Tuesday afternoon for her laryngitis (555-1632) – Dr. Findlay.				
	• Ross Muir is having marital problems and would like a counselling session on Wednesday after 2 p.m. (555-6741) – Dr. Cameron.				

		For Student's use		For Instructors use	
Task	**Instructions - Project 2**	**Yes**	**No**	**Errors**	**Total**
	INCOMING APPOINTMENT REQUESTS				
	• Jason Zabisewski (555-6522) needs appointment with Dr. Findlay on Wednesday morning – annual health exam for his twin daughters, Meredith and Paige.				
	• Mrs. Duncan requests an annual health exam with immunization for Elise (555-9359) Thursday morning appointment with Dr. Findlay.				
	• Lisa MacKenzie (555-0393), called in to cancel her Wednesday appointment. Did not rebook.				
	• Hope Gardner, R.N., calls from Strone Nursing Home requesting that Dr. Findlay visit Deirdre Sutherland on Wednesday afternoon as patient presents with onset of leg ulcer.				
	• Michael VanBerkel (555-2621) diabetic recheck early Wednesday afternoon – Dr. Cameron.				
	• Brandy Klein (555-8945) requests 9 o'clock appointment on Wednesday to see Dr. Findlay about her asthma.				
	• Kenneth Roberts (555-1481) preoperative checkup Wednesday afternoon with Dr. Cameron.				
	• Skye Hamilton (555-3906) 7-month prenatal checkup - Dr. Cameron, Friday morning.				

Instruction/Evaluation Sheet

TASK	INSTRUCTIONS - PROJECT 2	FOR STUDENT'S USE		FOR INSTRUCTORS USE	
		YES	NO	ERRORS	TOTAL
	INCOMING APPOINTMENT REQUESTS				
	• Jean Lewis (555-3254) would like an early Wednesday morning appointment with Dr. Findlay regarding intermittent dermatitis.				
	• Ewan Boyd – follow-up re foot x-ray (555-3807) would like appointment with Dr. Cameron on Friday after 2 p.m.				
	• William Alexander (555-4842) needs a prescription refill – Dr. Findlay, Wednesday.				
	• Hans Von Schroeder left a message cancelling his Friday appointment.				
	• Marshall Burns (555-6408) swollen elbow – Dr. Cameron on Wednesday.				
	• Mrs Fraser (555-4418) would like an annual health exam with immunization for Morag on Wednesday – Dr. Cameron.				
4	Prepare next day's day sheets for Dr. Cameron and Dr. Findlay. A sample is provided for your information.				

FOR PROFESSOR'S USE ONLY

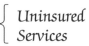
~~FEES FOR FORMS~~

Ontario Automobile Insurance Medical or Psychological Report
MVA Form 4, No Fault Benefits Schedule [*] $57.50

Driver Medical Examination (MOT) ~~FLRG80~~ $20.00 *$30*

~~Pilots Licence Validation Certificate, 26-005 (01-91)~~ .... ~~$20.00~~

~~Pilots Civil Aviation Examination Report, 26-0010 (0890)~~ .... ~~$50.00~~

School Physicals (Form) .... $15.00 ✓

Camp Physicals (Form) .... $15.00 ✓

Sick Notes .... $10.00 ✓

Back-to-Work Notes .... $10.00 ✓

Pre-Employment Certificate of Fitness .... $20.00 ✓

CPP Disability Medical Report, ~~ISP2519 (01/91)~~ .... $65.00 ✓

EI ~~UIC~~ Disability or Maternity Certificate ~~INS2019~~ .... $15.00 ✓

Daycare Notes ~~to verify free of communicable disease~~ .... $10.00 ✓

Medical Report for Canadian Immigrants .... ~~$25.00~~ ✓ *$40*

Hospital Employee Physicals .... $20.00 ✓

Revenue Canada, Federal Disability Tax Credit .... $20.00 ✓

Private Insurance, <u>s</u>ickness <u>f</u>orms .... ~~$22.30~~ *$22*

Private Insurance, <u>d</u>isability <u>f</u>orms .... ~~$22.30~~ *$22*

Private Insurance, <u>m</u>edical $50.00

OMA FEES FOR CONSULTATIONS AND VISITS

Consultation .... ~~76.60~~ *$79*

General Assessment .... ~~$71.90~~ *$75*

Intermediate Assessment .... ~~$36.95~~ *$39*

Minor Assessment .... ~~$24.25~~ *$25*

Annual Health Examination – <u>c</u>hild <u>a</u>fter Second <u>b</u>irthday .... ~~$41.45~~ *$43*

Prescription Renewals by Telephone $15.00

Transfer of Files $20.00-50.00

---

[*]The physician may consider charging a higher fee for cases whose complexity is greater than usual.

DAY SHEET EXAMPLE

DAY SHEET—MORNING

DR. CRAIG CAMERON   **Monday, August 28, 200X**

	PATIENT	REASON FOR APPOINTMENT	BILLING CODE	DIAGNOSIS
9:00				
9:15				
9:30				
9:45				
10:00	Sandra Armstrong	Annual Health Exam		
10:15				
10:30	COFFEE/MESSAGES			
10:45	Colin Blair	Ankle sprain		
11:00				
11:15	Ross Muir Scott Robinson	Tetanus/Polio injection Recheck blood pressure		
11:30	Barbara Urquhart	1st Obstetrical Visit		
11:45				
12:00	LUNCH			
12:15				
12:30				
12:45				
Remarks				

Argyll Clinic

PROJECT 3

NAME _____   DATE _____

TASK	INSTRUCTIONS - PROJECT 3	FOR STUDENT'S USE		FOR INSTRUCTOR'S USE	
		YES	NO	ERRORS	TOTAL
1	After returning telephone messages this morning, several patients require appointments today. (Refer to the following after hours telephone messages). Make the necessary changes to the Appointment Book and adjust the Day Sheets accordingly.				
2	Prepare charts for two new patients who will be seeing Dr. Cameron. Please refer to the sample patient chart provided. ■ The completed Patient Information Label should be affixed to the outside of the chart. ■ Affix a file folder label and alpha, colour-coded, peel-off tabs to the side of the chart. ■ Place index tabs on the folder dividers (yellow = x-ray, blue = lab reports, green = correspondence) and insert them in the chart. ■ Affix the Patient Summary to the inside front cover. ■ Place the Periodic Health Review and Clinical Data sheets in front of the folder dividers. ■ Attach the Patient Registration Form to the back inside cover of each the file folder.				
3	We have received relevant correspondence and reports from both patients' previous doctors. Correctly file this documentation in chronological order behind the appropriate dividers in each folder.				

Instruction/Evaluation Sheet

| TASK | INSTRUCTIONS - PROJECT 3 | FOR STUDENT'S USE | | FOR INSTRUCTOR'S USE | |
		YES	NO	ERRORS	TOTAL
	AFTER HOURS TELEPHONE MESSAGES				
	• Claire Nicholson (555-8069) needs counselling re her husband's drinking and physical abuse - Dr. Findlay				
	• Lindsay Wilson (555-0261) has painful lump in the armpit. She seemed very distressed - Dr. Cameron				
	• Mr. Shearlaw's son, Craig, to see Dr. Findlay about a swollen ankle from a tackle at a soccer game (555-9733)				
	• Iain Scott (555-7718) allergic reaction to insect bite - Dr. Cameron				
	• Robert Beattie has earache - Dr. Findlay (555-9547)				
	• Fiona Kerr (555-6940) has severe sunburn - Dr. Cameron				
	• Rhona Cairns (555-8174) UTI - Dr. Findlay				
	• Julie Burns (555-6436) vaginitis - Dr. Cameron				

FOR PROFESSOR'S USE ONLY

Patient Registration Forms

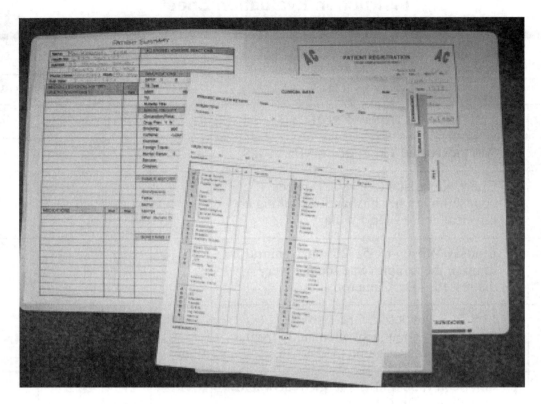

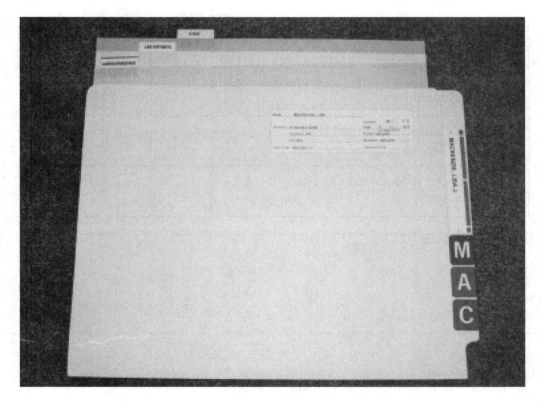

Patient Registration Forms

PATIENT REGISTRATION
(TO BE COMPLETED BY PATIENT)

Please Print

Please Check
Mr. □   Mrs. □   Miss □   Ms. ☑

LAST NAME: COLANGELO   FIRST NAME: ANITA

DATE OF BIRTH: DAY: 14   MONTH: January   YEAR: 1945

HEALTH CARD NUMBER: 7777-777-777   VERSION CODE: _____

TELEPHONE (HOME): 555-1314   (BUSINESS): 555-1632

ADDRESS: 463 Vistaview Road

CITY: Toronto   PROVINCE: ON   POSTAL CODE: F6Z 3L5

---- ✂ ---------- ✂ ----

PATIENT REGISTRATION
(TO BE COMPLETED BY PATIENT)

Please Print

Please Check
Mr. ☑   Mrs. □   Miss □   Ms. □

LAST NAME: VON SCHROEDER   FIRST NAME: HANS

DATE OF BIRTH: DAY: 1   MONTH: January   YEAR: 1940

HEALTH CARD NUMBER: 9999-999-999   VERSION CODE: _____

TELEPHONE (HOME): 555-9429   (BUSINESS): 555-1210

ADDRESS: 351 LONGMORE STREET

CITY: TORONTO   PROVINCE: ON   POSTAL CODE: F2X 2J5

Patient Information Labels

NAME _____

GENDER   M □   F □

ADDRESS _____

DOB ____/____/____

DAY/MONTH/YEAR

_____

PHONE _____

_____

BUSINESS _____

HEALTH NO _____

VERSION CODE _____

- - - - - - - - - - ✂ - - - - - - - - - - - - - - - - ✂ - - - - - - - - -

NAME _____

GENDER   M □   F □

ADDRESS _____

DOB ____/____/____

DAY/MONTH/YEAR

_____

PHONE _____

_____

BUSINESS _____

HEALTH NO _____

VERSION CODE _____

- - - - - - - - - - ✂ - - - - - - - - - - - - - - - - ✂ - - - - - - - - -

NAME _____

G   M □   F □

ADDRESS _____

DOB ____/____/____

DAY/MONTH/YEAR

_____

PHONE _____

_____

BUSINESS _____

HEALTH NO _____

VERSION CODE _____

- - - - - - - - - - ✂ - - - - - - - - - - - - - - - - ✂ - - - - - - - - -

NAME _____

GENDER   M □   F □

ADDRESS _____

DOB ____/____/____

DAY/MONTH/YEAR

_____

PHONE _____

_____

BUSINESS _____

HEALTH NO _____

VERSION CODE _____

Strathclyde Medical Laboratories

SML

456 Boswell Avenue
Toronto, ON F3L 5X5

☎ 555-1210
Result Reporting 555-1311

NAME: Anita Colangelo

DATE OF SERVICE: 08 May 2001

HEALTH NO: 7777 777 777

PCP: Dr. Neil Ferguson

DOB: 14 January 1945

SEX: F

TEST NAME	RESULT	ATTENTION	REFERENCE RANGE	UNITS
CYTOLOGY				
SOURCE		CERVIX		
CLINICAL DATA				
DATE OF LMP		NONE GIVEN		
MENOPAUSE?		NO		
PREGNANT?		NO		
BLEEDING?		NO		
DISCHARGE?		NO		
HORMONES?		NO		
RADIATION OR SURGERY?		NO		
PREVIOUS ATYP SMEARS:		NO OTHER DATA GIVEN		

****

PAP SMEAR

*ATYPCIAL SQUAMOUS CELLS OF UNDETERMINED SIGNIFICANCE. LOW GRADE SQUAMOUS INTRAEPITHELIAL LESION CANNOT BE EXCLUDED. SATISFACTORY FOR EVALUATION - TRANSFORMATION ZONE COMPONENT INCLUDED.
ENDOMETRIAL CELLS PRESENT.
**SUGGEST REPEAT SMEAR IN 6 MONTHS. INITIAL SCREENING WAS DONE AT HOLYROOD MEMORIAL HOSPITAL IN BALMORAL.

****

CYTOTECHNOLOGIST   MG
PATHOLOGIST   CASE REVIEWED BY RODERICK MACPHEE, MD

Strathclyde Medical Laboratories

456 Boswell Avenue
Toronto, ON F3L 5X5

☎ 555-1210
Result Reporting 555-1311

NAME: Hans Von Schroeder   **DATE OF SERVICE:** 26 Mar 2001   **HEALTH NO:** 9999 999 999

PCP: Dr. Andrew Rankin   **DOB:** 01 January 1940   **SEX:** M

TEST NAME	RESULT	ATTENTION	REFERENCE RANGE	UNITS
CHEMISTRY				
GLUCOSE FASTING		12.4 HI	3.3-6.1	MMOL/L
CREATININE	88		60-127	UMOL/L
URATE	404		180-450	UMOL/L
SODIUM		134	135-146	MMOL/L
POTASSIUM	4.4		3.7-5.4	MMOL/L
CHLORIDE	95		95-108	MMOL/L

Strathclyde Medical Laboratories

SML

456 Boswell Avenue
Toronto, ON F3L 5X5

☎ 555-1210
Result Reporting 555-1311

NAME: Anita Colangelo   **DATE OF SERVICE:** 13 June 2000   **HEALTH NO:** 7777 777 777

PCP: Dr. Neil Ferguson   **DOB:** 14 January 1945   **SEX:** F

TEST NAME	RESULT	ATTENTION	REFERENCE RANGE	UNITS
CHLAMYDIA				
SOURCE		CERVIX		
CHLAMYDIA		NEGATIVE		

Strathclyde Medical Laboratories

SML

456 Boswell Avenue
Toronto, ON F3L 5X5

☏ 555-1210
Result Reporting 555-1311

NAME: Anita Colangelo

PCP: Dr. Neil Ferguson

DATE OF SERVICE: 14 June 2000

DOB: 14 January 1945

HEALTH NO: 7777 777 777

SEX: F

TEST NAME	RESULT	ATTENTION	REFERENCE RANGE	UNITS
RIA				
TEST	1.67		0.30-4.70	MU/L

Strathclyde Medical Laboratories

456 Boswell Avenue
Toronto, ON F3L 5X5

S   555-1210
Result Reporting 555-1311

NAME: Anita Colangelo	**DATE OF SERVICE: 27 April 1999**	**HEALTH NO: 7777 777 777**
PCP: Dr. Neil Ferguson	**DOB: 14 January 1945**	**SEX: F**

TEST NAME	RESULT	ATTENTION	REFERENCE RANGE	UNITS

HISTORY

Wart left nostril

GROSS:

The specimen consists of a 0.4-cm fragment of tan tissue submitted in toto.

MICRO & DIAGNOSIS:

BIOPSY OF SKIN (LEFT NOSTRIL):
SUPERFICIAL FRAGMENTS OF SKIN WITH CHANGES OF
VERRUCA VULGARIS, BENIGN

RODERICK MACPHEE, M.D., B.Sc., F.R.C.P.(C)

Strathclyde Medical Laboratories

SML

456 Boswell Avenue
Toronto, ON F3L 5X5

☎ 555-1210
Result Reporting 555-1311

NAME: Anita Colangelo

DATE OF SERVICE: 28 Nov 2001

HEALTH NO: 7777 777 777

PCP: Dr. Neil Ferguson

DOB: 14 January 1945

SEX: F

TEST NAME	RESULT	ATTENTION	REFERENCE RANGE	UNITS
CHEMISTRY				
GLUCOSE FASTING	5.1		3.3-6.1	MMOL/L
CREATININE	74		60-115	UMOL/L
CHOLESTEROL	4.50		BELOW 5.20	MMOL/L
TRIGLYCERIDES	1.79		BELOW 2.30	MMOL/L
HDL CHOLESTEROL	1.20		0.90-2.07	MMOL/L
LDL CHOLESTEROL	2.49		BELOW 3.40	MMOL/L
LDL/HDL RATIO	2.08		BELOW 3.20	
CHOL/HDL RATIO	3.75		BELOW 4.40	

Strathclyde Medical Laboratories

456 Boswell Avenue
Toronto, ON F3L 5X5

☎ 555-1210
Result Reporting 555-1311

NAME: Hans Von Schroeder   **DATE OF SERVICE:** 12 Feb 2001   **HEALTH NO:** 9999 999 999

PCP: Dr. Andrew Rankin   **DOB:** 1 January, 1940   **SEX:** M

TEST NAME	RESULT	ATTENTION	REFERENCE RANGE	UNITS
HEMATOLOGY				
HEMOGLOBIN	141		115-165	G/L
HEMATOCRIT	0.410		0.37-0.47	L/L
WBC COUNT	7.9		4.0-11.0	X10 9L
RBC COUNT	4.63		3.80-5.80	X10-12L
MCV	88.6		80-97	FL
MCH	30.5		27.0-32.0	PG
MCHC	343		320-360	G/L
RDW	13.0		11.0-14.5	%
PLATELET COUNT	294		150-400	X10 9/L
ABSOLUTE: NEUTROS	4.2		2.0-7.5	X10 9/L
(A) LYMPH	3.0		1.1-3.3	X10 9/L
(A) MONO	0.5		0.0-0.8	X10 9/L
(A) EOS	0.1		0.0-0.5	X10 9/L
(A) BASO	0.0		0.0-0.2	X10 9/L
RBC MORPHOLOGY	NORMAL			
PLATELETS	NORMAL			

Strathclyde Medical Laboratories

SML

456 Boswell Avenue
Toronto, ON F3L 5X5

☎ 555-1210
Result Reporting 555-1311

NAME: Hans Von Schroeder   **DATE OF SERVICE:** 16 Apr 2001   **HEALTH NO:** 9999 999 999

PCP: Dr. Andrew Rankin   **DOB:** 01 January 1940   **SEX:** M

TEST NAME	RESULT	ATTENTION	REFERENCE RANGE	UNITS
HEMATOLOGY				
HEMOGLOBIN	161		115-165	G/L
HEMATOCRIT	0.466		0.37-0.47	L/L
WBC COUNT	9.1		4.0-11.0	X10 9L
RBC COUNT	5.17		3.80-5.80	X10-12L X10 9/L
MCV	89.9		80-97	FL
MCH	31.1		27.0-32.0	PG
MCHC	345		320-360	G/L
RDW	13.2		11.0-14.5	%
PLATELET COUNT	227		150-400	X10 9/L
ABSOLUTE: NEUTROS	5.9		2.0-7.5	X10 9/L
(A) LYMPH	2.4		1.1-3.3	X10 9/L
(A) MONO	0.6		0.0-0.8	X10 9/L
(A) EOS	0.2		0.0-0.5	X10 9/L
(A) BASO	0.0		0.0-0.2	X10 9/L
RBC MORPHOLOGY	NORMAL			
PLATELETS	NORMAL			
CHEMISTRY				
GLUCOSE FASTING		13.3 HI	3.3-6.1	MMOL/L
2 HR. P.C.		8.5 HI	3.6-7.8	MMOL/L
CREATININE	92		60-127	UMOL/L
SODIUM	137		135-146	MMOL/L
POTASSIUM	4.5		3.7-5.4	MMOL/L
ALK PHOS		130 HI	30-110	U/L

	NOTE: NEW REFERENCE RANGE			
AST	19		6-42	U/L
HEMOGLOBIN A1C		0.096	.045-.063	
CHOLESTEROL	2.77		BELOW 5.20	MMOL/L
TRIGLYCERIDES	1.00		BELOW 2.30	MMOL/L
HDL CHOLESTEROL		0.72	0.77-1.68	MMOL/L
LDL CHOLESTEROL	1.60		BELOW 3.40	MMOL/L
LDL HDL RATIO	2.22		BELOW 3.60	
CHOL/HDL RATIO	3.85		BELOW 5.00	
RIA				
TSH	0.58		0.30-4.70	MU/L

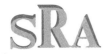 **STIRLING RADIOLOGICAL ASSOCIATES**

86 STIRLING ROAD, TORONTO, ON F2L 3X8
TEL: 555-5433
FAX: 555 3345

J.D. HALLIDAY, W.N. BRUCE, M.A. LEWIS
RADIOLOGISTS

Dr. Andrew Rankin
1281 Lochinvar Crescent
Perth, ON
F2G 3V5

Mr. Hans Von Schroeder
351 Longmore Street
Toronto, Ontario
F2X 2J5
555-9429
DOB: 1 January 1940

File Number: 285711
Visit Date: 04 November 1998

CHEST – PA AND LATERAL

The heart and mediastinum have a normal configuration for the age of the patient.
No skeletal lesions are seen.
The lungs and pleura are unremarkable.

OPINION: NO ACTIVE DISEASE

W.N. Bruce

W.N. Bruce, MD, FRCPC

DICTATED: 04.11.1998
TRANSCRIBED: 04.11.1998

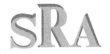
Dr. Neil Ferguson   Anita Colangelo
483 Blairmore Avenue   463 Vistaview Road
Selkirk, ON   Toronto, Ontario
F4L K3K   F6Z 3L5
                                           555-1314
                                           DOB: 14 January 1945

                                           File Number: 411356
                                           Visit Date: 10 August 2000

CHEST PA AND LATERAL

The heart size is within normal limits. There is slight unfolding of the aorta.
There are a few linear streaks in the right middle lobe area probably due to old
scarring; however, we have no previous film for comparison.

The lungs are otherwise clear.

J.D. Halliday

J.D. Halliday, MD, FRCPC

DICTATED: 10/08/2000
TRANSCRIBED: 11/08/2000

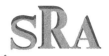 **STIRLING RADIOLOGICAL ASSOCIATES**

86 STIRLING ROAD, TORONTO, ON F2L 3X8
TEL: 555-5433
FAX: 555 3345

J.D. HALLIDAY, W.N. BRUCE, M.A. LEWIS
RADIOLOGISTS

Dr. Andrew Rankin
1281 Lochinvar Crescent
Perth, ON
F2G 3V5

Mr. Hans Von Schroeder
351 Longmore Street
Toronto, Ontario
FX 2J5
555-9429
DOB: 1 January 1940

File Number: 421210
Visit Date: 08 December 2000

BOTH KNEES

There is moderate spurring of the tibial spines of both knees, and there is minor lipping around the medial and lateral compartments. There is minimal patellofemoral joint OA. No joint space narrowing is seen.

J.D. Halliday

J.D. Halliday, MD, FRCPC

DICTATED: 08/12/2000
TRANSCRIBED: 09/12/2000

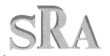 **STIRLING RADIOLOGICAL ASSOCIATES**

86 STIRLING ROAD, TORONTO, ON F2L 3X8   J.D. HALLIDAY, W.N. BRUCE, M.A. LEWIS
TEL: 555-5433   RADIOLOGISTS
FAX: 555 3345

Dr. Neil Ferguson
483 Blairmore Avenue
Selkirk, ON
F4L K3K

Anita Colangelo
463 Vistaview Road
Toronto, Ontario
F6Z 3L5
555-1314
DOB: 14 January 1945

File Number: 393717
Visit Date: 23 December 1999

BILATERAL MAMMOGRAM

There is no evidence of malignancy. No significant abnormality is seen.

J.D. Halliday, MD, FRCPC

DICTATED: 23/12/1999
TRANSCRIBED: 23/12/1999

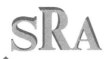

STIRLING RADIOLOGICAL ASSOCIATES

86 STIRLING ROAD, TORONTO, ON F2L 3X8
TEL: 555-5433
FAX: 555 3345

J.D. HALLIDAY, W.N. BRUCE, M.A. LEWIS
RADIOLOGISTS

Dr. Andrew Rankin
1281 Lochinvar Crescent
Perth, ON
F2G 3V5

Mr. Hans Von Schroeder
351 Longmore Street
Toronto, Ontario
F2X 2J5
555-9429
DOB: 1 January 1940

File Number: 423681
Visit Date: 27 November 2000

CHEST PA AND LATERAL

The mediastinum and cardiac silhouette are normal in size and contour. There is hyperinflation of the lungs, with prominence of the right basalar bronchovascular markings, all in keeping with chronic obstructive pulmonary disease. There is, however, no pneumonia.

W.N. Bruce, MD, FRCPC

DICTATED: 30 November 2000
TRANSCRIBED: 30 November 2000

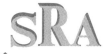 **STIRLING RADIOLOGICAL ASSOCIATES**

86 STIRLING ROAD, TORONTO, ON F2L 3X8
TEL: 555-5433
FAX: 555 3345

J.D. HALLIDAY, W.N. BRUCE, M.A. LEWIS
RADIOLOGISTS

Dr. Andrew Rankin
1281 Lochinvar Crescent
Perth, ON
F2G 3V5

Mr. Hans Von Schroeder
351 Longmore Street
Toronto, Ontario
F2X 2J5
555-9429
DOB: 1 January 1940

File Number: 573697
Visit Date: 19 March 1998

LEFT SHOULDER

No bone or joint abnormality is seen and there is no soft tissue calcification.

M.A. Lewis, MD, FRCPC

DICTATED: 19 March 1998
TRANSCRIBED: 19 March 1998

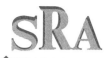

STIRLING RADIOLOGICAL ASSOCIATES

86 STIRLING ROAD, TORONTO, ON F2L 3X8
TEL: 555-5433
FAX: 555 3345

J.D. HALLIDAY, W.N. BRUCE, M.A. LEWIS
RADIOLOGISTS

Dr. Neil Ferguson
483 Blairmore Avenue
Selkirk, ON
F4L K3K

Anita Colangelo
463 Vistaview Road
Toronto, Ontario
F6Z 3L5
555-1314
DOB: 1 4 January 1945

File Number: 436579
Visit Date: 17 March 2001

ABDOMINAL ULTRASOUND

No calculi are seen in the gallbladder. The ducts are normal. No abnormality is seen in the liver, spleen, pancreas, aorta, or kidneys.

J.D. HALLIDAY, MD, FRCPC

DICTATED: 17 March 2001
TRANSCRIBED: 17 March 2001

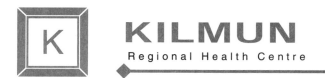

KILMUN
Regional Health Centre

15 Graham's Point
Toronto, ON F9L 1S5

December 18, 2001

Dr. Andrew Rankin
1281 Lochinvar Crescent
Toronto, ON F2G 3V5

Dear Dr. Rankin

Re: Hans Von Schroeder

Thank you for referring this pleasant gentleman to me.

Mr. Von Schroeder advised me that approximately eighteen months ago he developed an itchy rash on the trunk, arms, and in the groin area. There has been some improvement following the use of Lotriderm cream, but he still has intermittent activity in the groin and now in the perianal area. A few months ago, he developed an itchy rash on the lower limbs, but this has improved considerably with the use of Elocom cream.

Examination revealed slight erythema in the groin folds and in the perianal area. This is most likely seborrheic dermatitis. If possible, I would like to control this with a low potency topical steroid. I have asked him to slowly reduce the use of Lotriderm cream and instead to use Desocort cream and Nizoral cream, each applied b.i.d.

He also has a mild dermatitis on the lower legs. This is clearly under very good control with Elocom cream, which I have asked him to continue.

I have asked this patient to see me again in three weeks if his symptoms do not improve. Thank you for your referral of this patient.

Yours sincerely

Carolynn Young

Carolynn Young, MD, FRCPC

CY/ne

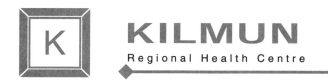

KILMUN

Regional Health Centre

15 Graham's Point
Toronto, ON F9L 1S5

December 5, 2001

Dr. Andrew Rankin
1281 Lochinvar Crescent
Toronto, ON F2G 3V5

Dear Dr. Rankin

Re: Hans Von Schroeder

Hans was in to see me today, and I am happy to report that the ulcer on the dorsal aspect of his right foot is healing nicely. At the present time, there is no more undermining, and we can now expect to see a gradual reduction in the diameter of the lesion.

Hans has noticed a marked decrease of the discomfort and is quite happy with his progress. I will see him again early in the New Year.

Yours truly

Heather Buchanan, MD, FRCSC

HB/ams

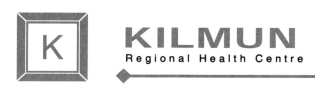

May 20, 2002

Dr. Neil Ferguson
483 Blairmore Avenue
Toronto, ON F4L K3K

Dear Dr. Ferguson:

Re: Anita Colangelo

Anita was in my office today to discuss her progress. It is now two months since I biopsied the lesion of the right cheek and shaved the nevus from the right alar dome. The cheek lesion has been diagnosed as a benign compound nevus.

The nasal tip shows slight indentation where the lesion was removed, but it is gradually improving, and I have advised Anita to give it at least another three months for further maturation.

Yours truly,

Gordon J. Dingwall, M.D., F.R.C.S. (C.)

GJD/yi

Patient Summary

Name	ALLERGIES/ADVERSE REACTIONS
Health No	
Address	
Phone: Home Work	
Date of Birth	IMMUNIZATIONS

MEDICAL AND SURGICAL HISTORY HEALTH CONDITIONS

HEALTH CONDITIONS	Date

IMMUNIZATIONS				
DPTP 1	2	3	4	5
TB Test				
MMR Hib				
Td				
Rubella Titre				

FAMILY HISTORY

Grandparents

Father

Mother

Siblings

Other (Genetic Disorders, Risk Factors)

SOCIAL HISTORY

Marital Status: S   M   CL   Sep   Div   W

Spouse

Children

Occupation/Risks

Drug Plan: Yes ®   No ®

Smoking: ppd

Caffeine: cups/day   Alcohol: oz/wk

Exercise

Foreign Travel

SCREENING/PREVENTION

MEDICATIONS

MEDICATIONS	Start	Stop

Patient Summary

Name	ALLERGIES/ADVERSE REACTIONS
Health No	
Address	
Phone: Home Work	
Date of Birth	

<table>
<tr><td colspan="2">MEDICAL AND SURGICAL HISTORY
HEALTH CONDITIONS</td><td>Date</td></tr>
</table>

IMMUNIZATIONS

DPTP	1	2	3	4	5
TB Test					
MMR	Hib				
Td					
Rubella Titre					

FAMILY HISTORY

Grandparents
Father
Mother
Siblings
Other (Genetic Disorders, Risk Factors)

SOCIAL HISTORY

Marital Status: S   M   CL   Sep   Div   W
Spouse
Children
Occupation/Risks
Drug Plan: Yes ®   No ®
Smoking: ppd
Caffeine: cups/day   Alcohol: oz/wk
Exercise
Foreign Travel

MEDICATIONS	Start	Stop

SCREENING/PREVENTION

Periodic Health Review

Name _____ **Age** _____ **Date** _____

SUBJECTIVE

Problems: 1. _____ 2. _____ 3. _____

_____

_____

_____

_____

OBJECTIVE

Wt: _____ **Ht:** _____ **BP: L** _____ **BP: R** _____ **HR** _____ **RR** _____ **T** _____

Appearance: _____ **Urine:** _____

		N	A	Remarks			N	A	Remarks
HEAD AND NECK	Visual Acuity Conj/Scler/Lids Pupils: light accom. Fundi Ears Nose/Sinuses Throat Teeth/Gums Cervical Nodes Thyroid			L ____ R ____	**GENITOURINARY**	Vulva Vagina Cervix Pap performed Uterus Adnexae Prolapse Penis Testes Prostate	Y	N	
CHEST	Inspection Auscultation Breasts Axillary Nodes				**MSK**	Spine Extrem: bony s.tis. Joints			
CVS	Heart Sounds Murmurs Carotid Bruits JVP Pulses: fem p.tib. d.ped. Edema Varicose Veins				**NEUROLOGIC**	Mental Status Cranial Nerves Motor: bulk tone power ab.mvmt. Sensation Reflexes Co-ordination Gait			
ABDOMEN	Contour BS Masses Tender L/S/K/K Ing. Nodes Hernia Rectal				**SKIN**	Scalp/Hair Nails Lesions Nevi			

Assessment

_____

_____

_____

Plan

_____

_____

_____

Periodic Health Review

Name _____ **Age** _____ **Date** _____

SUBJECTIVE

Problems: 1. _____ 2. _____ 3. _____

_____
_____
_____
_____

OBJECTIVE

Wt: _____ Ht: _____ BP: L _____ BP: R _____ HR _____ RR _____ T _____

Appearance: _____ Urine: _____

		N	A	Remarks			N	A	Remarks
HEAD AND NECK	Visual Acuity Conj/Scler/Lids Pupils: light accom. Fundi Ears Nose/Sinuses Throat Teeth/Gums Cervical Nodes Thyroid			L ____ R ____	**GENITOURINARY**	Vulva Vagina Cervix Pap performed Uterus Adnexae Prolapse Penis Testes Prostate	Y	N	
CHEST	Inspection Auscultation Breasts Axillary Nodes				**MSK**	Spine Extrem: bony s.tis. Joints			
CVS	Heart Sounds Murmurs Carotid Bruits JVP Pulses: fem p.tib. d.ped. Edema Varicose Veins				**NEUROLOGIC**	Mental Status Cranial Nerves Motor: bulk tone power ab.mvmt. Sensation Reflexes Co-ordination Gait			
ABDOMEN	Contour BS Masses Tender L/S/K/K Ing. Nodes Hernia Rectal				**SKIN**	Scalp/Hair Nails Lesions Nevi			

Assessment

_____
_____
_____

Plan

_____
_____
_____

Clinical Data

Name _____ **DOB** _____ **Page** __

Clinical Data

Name _____ **DOB** _____ **Page** _____

Argyll Clinic

PROJECT 4

NAME _____   **DATE** _____

TASK	INSTRUCTIONS - PROJECT 4	FOR STUDENT'S USE		FOR INSTRUCTOR'S USE	
		YES	NO	ERRORS	TOTAL
1	Create Dr. Durrant's appointment schedule for Friday using appointment scheduling software. Dr. Durrant prefers to have his appointments scheduled using the computerized appointment software; therefore, input the patient information and prepare and print out a copy of Friday's day sheet.				
	PATIENT NAME AND REASON FOR APPOINTMENT				
	Your Name Acne				
	Lisa MacKenzie Diarrhea				
	Lindsay Wilson Constipation				
	Fiona Kerr Sore wrist				
	Julie Burns CPX & pap smear				
	Rhona Cairns Low back pain				
	Sandra Armstrong Contraceptive advice				
	Barbara Urquhart Cellulitis				
	Colin Blair Duodenal ulcer				

TASK	INSTRUCTIONS - PROJECT 4	FOR STUDENT'S USE		FOR INSTRUCTOR'S USE	
		YES	NO	ERRORS	TOTAL
	PATIENT NAME AND REASON FOR APPOINTMENT (continued)				
	Iain Scott Annual health examination				
	Scott Robinson Gout				
	Marshall Burns Follow-up re rest results				
	Ross Muir Tendonitis				
	Elise Duncan Wart treatment				
	Skye Hamilton Dermatitis				
2	In addition to physician services, Argyll Clinic provides ultrasound examinations and x-rays. The ultrasound technician has asked you to create the attached fill-in form as a template, using the Argyll letterhead.				
	• Assess the form and determine the appropriate form fields to be used and incorporate the handwritten instructions.				
	• Save the form as **Diagnostic Imaging** on your disk, print a copy, and close the template.				

DIAGNOSTIC ULTRASOUND CONSULTATION REQUEST

Name:

Address

Telephone No:

Date of Birth

MOH Number

APPOINTMENT DATE   TIME:

EXAMINATION REQUESTED

☐ Gallbladder   ☐ Pelvis

☐ Liver   ☐ Obstetrics

☐ Pancreas   ☐ Aorta

☐ Kidney   ⬚   ◄— *drop down*   ☐ Other
                              { *Left*
                              { *Right*

CLINICAL INFORMATION

Prior x-ray or ultrasound examination

Kilmun Reg. Health Centre   ☐ No   ☐ Yes   Date

Other Location   ☐ No   ☐ Yes   Date

Physician's signature: _____

   Current Date: _____

		FOR STUDENT'S USE		FOR INSTRUCTOR'S USE	
TASK	INSTRUCTIONS - PROJECT 4	YES	NO	ERRORS	TOTAL
3	Fill in the newly created form template for patient Anita Colangelo using the following data:				
	• The 18 of next month, current year at 8:30 a.m. • Left kidney • Clinic info – N/A • Previous exam at Kilmun - No • Other location - Yes - June 4 last year				
	• Save the filled-in form as **Colangelo** and print one copy				
4	Input the following form letter using Argyll letterhead, and mail out to patients as per instructions.				
	• Use full-block letter style with open punctuation.				
	• Save the form letter as **diabetes** and print a copy				
	• Save the variable information (data source) as **diabetes data** and print a copy.				
	• Save the three merged documents as **diabetes merge** and print the merged letters.				
	• Information for the seminars is as follows: Scott Robinson October 17 at 6 p.m. Fiona Kerr October 24 at 8 p.m. Your Name November 5 at 6:30 p.m.				

<u>Diabetes Mellitus Seminar</u>

associated
Dr. Catharine Russell, who is ~~affiliated~~ with our clinic, plans to offer a ⟵ *stet*
series of four seminars for her diabetes mellitus patients and their spouses.

The purpose of these sessions is to educate patients and families on current methods of controlling diabetes. This informative seminar deals with ⟍ *run on*

How Diet and Exercise Contribute to the Well-being of Diabetes Patients.

Italics

Accordingly, you and your spouse are invited to attend a session to be held at our ~~office~~ on _____ at _____
clinic

Please telephone the clinic as soon as poss. to confirm your attendance

yt

CC

Instruction/Evaluation Sheet

TASK	INSTRUCTIONS - PROJECT 4	FOR STUDENT'S USE		FOR INSTRUCTOR'S USE	
		YES	NO	ERRORS	TOTAL
5	Correctly fill out a Physician Referral for Dr. Cameron's signature for Hans Von Schroeder to attend the Diabetes Clinic.				
	• Keep a copy of this form in the patient's chart				

FOR PROFESSOR'S USE ONLY

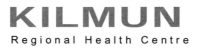

KILMUN
Regional Health Centre

15 Graham's Point
Toronto, ON F9L 1S5

For office use only

PHYSICIAN REFERRAL
Diabetes Clinic—Education
The Blairmore Mall
89 Gibb's Brae
Toronto, ON   F9L 1S3

REQUIRED INFORMATION

Name _____

Telephone: Home _____   Office _____

Date of Birth _____

Duration of Illness _____   BP _____

History of Illness _____

_____

MEDICATIONS—DIABETES

Hypoglycemic Agents—Oral _____   Date began _____

_____   Date began _____

Insulin _____   Date began _____

Any other Medicines _____

_____

LABORATORY RESULTS

FBS _____   2 hr. pc _____

HbA1C _____   (This information is required by the Ministry of Health and Long-term Care)

HDL _____   LDL _____   Total Cholesterol _____

TSH _____   Albumin/creatinine ratio _____

Triglycerides _____   Microalbuminuria _____

Prognosis _____

_____

By my signature below, the nurse is authorized to make minor adjustments to the above-named patient's insulin/oral diabetes medication in accordance with blood glucose meter results.   ☐ Yes   ☐ No

Referring doctor _____   Today's Date _____

Telephone _____   Fax _____

Please fax the completed form to the Diabetes Clinic—Education at 555 6741.

Argyll Clinic

PROJECT 5

NAME _____   DATE _____

TASK	INSTRUCTIONS - PROJECT 5	FOR STUDENT'S USE		FOR INSTRUCTOR'S USE	
		YES	NO	ERRORS	TOTAL
1	Using Argyll letterhead, transcribe the two letters on disk, using full block and open punctuation.				
	These documents must be ready for signature before the end of the day.				
	The first letter is to Dr. Daniel C. Reive, 810 Ferrier Boulevard, Toronto, F5T 3R7 from Dr. James Driuna. The patient's name is Amanda MacLean				
	The second letter is to Dr. Lorna D. Maxwell, 167 Bothwell Road, Toronto, ON F5T M8S from Dr. Arlene Baird. Patient's name is Douglas Graham.				
2	Using the Petty Cash Form, record the cash transactions for the month of August.				
	Aug 1 Opening Balance $150.00				
	3 Postage stamps $14.77				
	5 Coffee, tea, sugar, and milk $23.79				
	10 Post-it notes $5.50				
	12 Daily newspaper $1.50				
	16 Blair Couriers (specimens to Strathclyde Medical Lab) $8.80				
	19 Set of office keys cut at Ballantyne Locksmith $7.50				
	20 Paper clips $5.39				
	22 Pens $6.55				

| | | FOR STUDENT'S USE | | FOR INSTRUCTOR'S USE | |
| | | YES | NO | ERRORS | TOTAL |
TASK	**INSTRUCTIONS - PROJECT 5**	YES	NO	ERRORS	TOTAL
	Aug 27 Daily newspaper $1.50				
	30 Blair Couriers (disk to MOHLTC) $17.60				
	• Bank balance as at August 31 $8,725.31				
	• Determine the amount required to restore the petty cash fund to $150 as at August 31; write out a cheque for that amount.				
3	You were hired as a full-time medical administrative assistant for Argyll Clinic on August 21. Fill out the appropriate personal information on the Employee Payroll Record before you calculate your first pay. Prepare the payroll for both you and Julie Tassopoulos, using the Employee Payroll Records and Payroll Statements for the pay period ending September 1. Specific instructions are below.				
	• Calculate the gross pay (Total Earnings) for this pay period for Julie and you.				
	• Your rate of pay - $18 per hour • Hours worked - 70 hours this pay period (7-hour day, Monday through Friday)				
	• Julie's rate of pay - $13 per hour • Hours worked - 35 hours this pay period broken down as follows: Days Monday Wednesday Friday Hours 5 7.5 5 Hours 7.5 5 5				

TASK	INSTRUCTIONS - PROJECT 5	FOR STUDENT'S USE		FOR INSTRUCTOR'S USE	
		YES	NO	ERRORS	TOTAL
	• Use Federal and Provincial Tax Category 1 for both you and Julie.				
	• Calculate the net pay for one biweekly period (26 pay periods a year) using the *Payroll Deductions Tables*				
	• This period's pay date is Friday, September 1.				
	• Complete an Employee Payroll Statement for each of you.				
	• Write out the payroll cheques.				
4	Record the following transactions in the Cash Disbursements Journal. Consecutive cheques were issued for these expenditures, beginning with Cheque No. 176.				
	Aug 1 Argyll Professional Building (rent) $3500.00				
	4 Julie Tassopoulos (wages)				
	7 Gas Services (office heat) $146.29				
	7 Energy Hydro $61.15				
	8 Dunbar Records Imaging (conversion of inactive patient charts to a digital medium) $835.00				
	14 Clydesdale Medical Supplies (table paper and disposable needles) $78.00				
	14 Anderson Surgical Supply (gauze sponges, sterilizing solution, paper gowns) $325.46				
	14 Kirkpatrick Couriers (courier services) $15.38				
	14 Office Essentials (paper clips, pens, file folders) $223.00				

Instruction/Evaluation Sheet

		FOR STUDENT'S USE		FOR INSTRUCTOR'S USE	
TASK	**INSTRUCTIONS - PROJECT 5**	YES	NO	ERRORS	TOTAL
	Aug 18 Julie Tassopoulos - Wages				
	28 Marvelous Maintenance Services (office cleaning) $400.00				
	28 Dial Canada (telephone service) $109.33				
	28 Prompt Page (paging service) $45.67				
	28 Argyll Medical Pharmacy (medical supplies) $124.30				
	28 Bradley's Computer Company (computer supplies) $41.19				
	31 Reimburse petty cash				
	• Total and cross balance all applicable columns.				

FOR PROFESSOR'S USE ONLY

Petty Cash

Date	Particulars	Amount Paid Out	Newspapers Journals	Office Supplies	Courier	Postage	Misc.	Total
	Opening Balance							
	Column Totals							
	Amount to Replenish Fund							
	Balance Carried Forward							

EMPLOYEE PAYROLL RECORD

DETACH THIS SECTION AND PLACE IN EMPLOYEE'S PERSONNEL FILE FOR EASY REFERENCE

NAME: Julie Tassopoulos

EMPLOYEE EARNINGS																					
MONTH	WEEK ENDING	❶ DAILY HOURS							HOURS									❺ TOTAL HOURLY EARNINGS	❻ OTHER EARNINGS	❼ TOTAL EARNINGS	❽ TAXABLE BENEFITS
		S	M	T	W	T	F	S	❷ REG.	RATE	S-TOTAL	❸ × 1 1/2	RATE	S-TOTAL	❹ × 2	RATE	S-TOTAL				
JULY	7		4		6		4		28 h	13 00	364 00	h			h			364 00		364 00	
	14		5		5		5		h			h			h						
	21		5		5		5		30 h	13 00	390 00	h			h			390 00		390 00	
	28		5		4		4		h			h			h						
									h			h			h						
		JULY TOTALS:							58 h		754 00	h			h			754 00		754 00	
AUGUST	4		4		4		4		25 h	13 00	325 00	h			h			325 00		325 00	
	11		5		6		5		h			h			h						
	18		6		5		5		32 h	13 00	416 00	h			h			416 00		416 00	
	25								h			h			h						
									h			h			h						
		AUGUST TOTALS:							57 h		741 00	h			h			741 00		741 00	
SEPTEMBER	1								h			h			h						
	8								h			h			h						
	15								h			h			h						
	22								h			h			h						
	29								h			h			h						
		SEPTEMBER TOTALS:							h			h			h						
OCTOBER									h			h			h						
									h			h			h						
									h			h			h						
									h			h			h						
									h			h			h						
		OCTOBER TOTALS:							h			h			h						
NOVEMBER									h			h			h						
									h			h			h						
									h			h			h						
									h			h			h						
									h			h			h						
		NOVEMBER TOTALS:							h			h			h						
DECEMBER									h			h			h						
									h			h			h						
									h			h			h						
									h			h			h						
									h			h			h						
		DECEMBER TOTALS:							h			h			h						

DETACH AND DISPOSE

EMPLOYEE INFORMATION

NAME: JULIE		SIN 4|2|8|1|7|0|3|6|9	TYPE OF WORK	UNION RATE:	PENSION PLAN RATE:	WAGE RATES AND REVISIONS	
SURNAME: TASSOPOULOS		DATE OF BIRTH: 8|1|1|1|1|0		REFERENCE IN PAYROLL BOOK:		DATE	HOURLY / WEEKLY / OTHERS
ADDRESS: 126 FRONT ST	CITY: TORONTO	YEAR MONTH DAY	JOB CODE UNION	WEEKS OF		1/9/01	13.00
PROVINCE: ON POSTAL CODE: F6P 1X7 TEL: 555-6526 FAX:				VACATION			
LAST EMPLOYER: LAST OCCUPATION:		MALE ☐ FEMALE ☒	EXEMPTION CODE	EMPLOYMENT DATE YEAR 01 MONTH 09 DAY 01			
EDUCATION DEGREE: ADDITIONAL COURSES:			FEDERAL	TERMINATION DATE			
CIVIL STATUS: MARRIED OR EQUIVALENT ☐ DIVORCED ☐ WIDOW(ER) ☐ SINGLE ☒ NUMBER OF DEPENDENTS ☐			PROVINCIAL	DATE OF NOTICE	REASON:		

EMPLOYEE DEDUCTION / NET EARNINGS

⑨ TAX DEDUCTIBLE AMOUNT	⑩ TAXABLE EARNINGS	⑪ DED.	⑫ CUMUL.	⑬ INS. EARN	⑭ DED.	FEDERAL	PROVINCIAL	⑯ REG'D PENSION PLAN	⑰ UNION DUES	⑱ OTHER DEDUCTIONS	⑲ HEALTH INS.	⑳ GROUP INS.	㉑ OTHERS	㉒ TOTAL DEDUCTIONS	㉓ AMOUNT PAID	CHEQUE NO.	㉔ DATE	MONTH
	364 00	10 78	142 90	364 00	8 01	8 25								27 04	336 96	150	7/7	J U L Y
	390 00	12 00	154 90	390 00	8 58	11 85								32 43	357 57	157	21/7	
	754 00	22 78		754 00	16 59	20 10								59 47	694 53			
	325 00	8 95	163 85	325 00	7 15	2 30								18 40	306 60	177	4/8	A U G U S T
	416 00	13 23	177 08	416 00	9 15	16 00								38 38	377 62	185	18/8	
	741 00	22 18		741 00	16 30	18 30								56 78	684 22			
																		S E P T E M B E R
																		O C T O B E R
																		N O V E M B E R
																		D E C E M B E R
A																		
B																		
C																		

COMMENTS:

EMPLOYEE PAYROLL RECORD

DETACH THIS SECTION AND PLACE IN
EMPLOYEE'S PERSONNEL FILE FOR EASY REFERENCE

		EMPLOYEE EARNINGS													
MONTH	WEEK ENDING	❶ DAILY HOURS		HOURS									❺ TOTAL HOURLY EARNINGS	❻ OTHER EARNINGS	❼ TOTAL EARNINGS	❽ TAXABLE BENEFITS
		S M T W T F S	❷ REG.	RATE	S-TOTAL	❸ × 1½	RATE	S-TOTAL	❹ × 2	RATE	S-TOTAL				
J U L Y			h			h			h						
			h			h			h						
			h			h			h						
			h			h			h						
			h			h			h						
	JULY TOTALS:		h			h			h						
A U G U S T			h			h			h						
			h			h			h						
			h			h			h						
			h			h			h						
			h			h			h						
	AUGUST TOTALS:		h			h			h						
S E P T E M B E R			h			h			h						
			h			h			h						
			h			h			h						
			h			h			h						
			h			h			h						
	SEPTEMBER TOTALS:		h			h			h						
O C T O B E R			h			h			h						
			h			h			h						
			h			h			h						
			h			h			h						
			h			h			h						
	OCTOBER TOTALS:		h			h			h						
N O V E M B E R			h			h			h						
			h			h			h						
			h			h			h						
			h			h			h						
			h			h			h						
	NOVEMBER TOTALS:		h			h			h						
D E C E M B E R			h			h			h						
			h			h			h						
			h			h			h						
			h			h			h						
			h			h			h						
	DECEMBER TOTALS:		h			h			h						

DETACH AND DISPOSE

EMPLOYEE INFORMATION

NAME:		SIN								TYPE OF WORK	UNION RATE:	PENSION PLAN RATE:	WAGE RATES AND REVISIONS			
SURNAME:		DATE OF BIRTH:									REFERENCE IN PAYROLL BOOK:		DATE	HOURLY	WEEKLY	OTHERS
ADDRESS:	CITY:			YEAR MONTH DAY		JOB CODE	UNION	WEEKS OF						
PROVINCE:	POSTAL CODE:	TEL:	FAX:					VACATION						
LAST EMPLOYER:	LAST OCCUPATION:		MALE ☐ FEMALE ☐	EXEMPTION CODE		EMPLOYMENT DATE	YEAR MONTH DAY			
EDUCATION DEGREE:	ADDITIONAL COURSES:		FEDERAL		TERMINATION DATE				
CIVIL STATUS: MARRIED OR EQUIVALENT ☐ DIVORCED ☐ WIDOW(ER) ☐ SINGLE ☐ NUMBER OF DEPENDENTS ☐	PROVINCIAL		DATE OF NOTICE			REASON:			

EMPLOYEE DEDUCTION — NET EARNINGS

⑨ TAX DEDUCTIBLE AMOUNT	⑩ TAXABLE EARNINGS	GOVERNMENT PENSION PLAN		EMPLOYMENT INSURANCE		⑮ INCOME TAX		⑯ REG'D PENSION PLAN	⑰ UNION DUES	⑱ OTHER DEDUCTIONS	⑲ HEALTH INS.	⑳ GROUP INS.	㉑ OTHERS	㉒ TOTAL DEDUCTIONS	㉓ AMOUNT PAID	CHEQUE NO.	㉔ DATE	MONTH
		⑪ DED.	⑫ CUMUL.	⑬ INS. EARN	⑭ DED.	FEDERAL	PROVINCIAL											
																		J U L Y
																		A U G U S T
																		S E P T E M B E R
																		O C T O B E R
																		N O V E M B E R
																		D E C E M B E R
A																		
B																		
C																		

COMMENTS:

Employee Payroll Statement

EMPLOYER:

HOURS WORKED					WORK PERIOD WEEK ENDING		
	HOURS	RATE	SUB TOTAL		YEAR	MONTH	DAY
② REG.							
③ x 1 1/2							
④ x 2							

EARNINGS		DEDUCTIONS			
⑥ OTHER EARN.	⑤ TOTAL HOURLY EARNINGS	⑮ INCOME TAX	⑳ GROUP INSURANCE		
	⑦ TOTAL EARNINGS				
⑧ TAXABLE BEN.		⑯ REG'D PENSION PLAN	㉑ OTHERS		
⑩ TAXABLE EARNINGS		⑰ UNION DUES	⑨ TAX DED. AMOUNT		
⑪ GOVERNMENT PENSION PLAN		⑲ HEALTH INSURANCE	㉒ TOTAL DEDUCTIONS		
⑭ EMPLOYMENT INSURANCE					

NET EARNINGS

㉔ CHEQUE NO.	DATE	㉓ AMOUNT PAID

EMPLOYEE:

ADDRESS:

OCCUPATION:

EMPLOYER:

HOURS WORKED					WORK PERIOD WEEK ENDING		
	HOURS	RATE	SUB TOTAL		YEAR	MONTH	DAY
② REG.							
③ x 1 1/2							
④ x 2							

EARNINGS		DEDUCTIONS			
⑥ OTHER EARN.	⑤ TOTAL HOURLY EARNINGS	⑮ INCOME TAX	⑳ GROUP INSURANCE		
	⑦ TOTAL EARNINGS				
⑧ TAXABLE BEN.		⑯ REG'D PENSION PLAN	㉑ OTHERS		
⑩ TAXABLE EARNINGS		⑰ UNION DUES	⑨ TAX DED. AMOUNT		
⑪ GOVERNMENT PENSION PLAN		⑲ HEALTH INSURANCE	㉒ TOTAL DEDUCTIONS		
⑭ EMPLOYMENT INSURANCE					

NET EARNINGS

㉔ CHEQUE NO.	DATE	㉓ AMOUNT PAID

EMPLOYEE:

ADDRESS:

OCCUPATION:

ALL RIGHTS RESERVED © 1998, BLUELINE® EMPLOYEE PAYROLL STATEMENT A1000

Employee Payroll Statement Example

EMPLOYER: _XZ Company_

Anytown, Canada

WORK PERIOD		
WEEK ENDING		
YEAR	MONTH	DAY
20xx	01	08

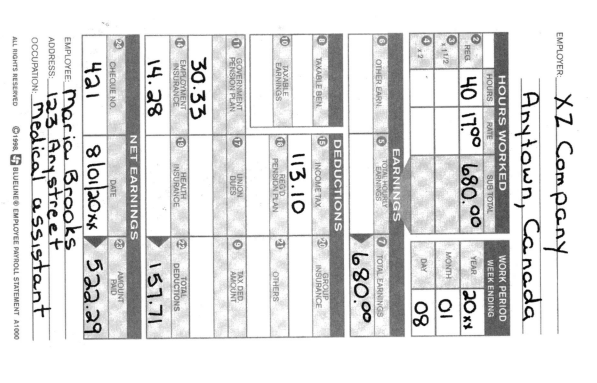

HOURS WORKED				EARNINGS					
	HOURS	RATE	SUB TOTAL						
② REG.	40	17.00	680.00						
③ x 1 1/2									
④ x 2									
				⑤ TOTAL HOURLY EARNINGS					
⑥ OTHER EARN.									
				⑥ TOTAL HOURLY EARNINGS	680.00			⑦ TOTAL EARNINGS	

DEDUCTIONS							
⑧ TAXABLE BEN.		⑮ INCOME TAX	113.10	⑳ GROUP INSURANCE			
⑩ TAXABLE EARNINGS		⑯ REG'D PENSION PLAN		㉑ OTHERS			
⑪ GOVERNMENT PENSION PLAN	30.33	⑰ UNION DUES		⑨ TAX DED. AMOUNT			
⑫ EMPLOYMENT INSURANCE	14.28	⑲ HEALTH INSURANCE		㉒ TOTAL DEDUCTIONS	157.71		

NET EARNINGS			
㉔ CHEQUE NO.	DATE		㉓ AMOUNT PAID
421	8 01 20xx		522.29

EMPLOYEE: _Maria Brooks_
ADDRESS: _123 Anystreet_
OCCUPATION: _Medical assistant_

Canada Pension Plan Contributions
Biweekly (26 pay periods a year)

Cotisations au Régime de pensions du Canada
Aux deux semaines (26 périodes de paie par année)

Pay Rémunération From - De	To - À	CPP RPC	Pay Rémunération From - De	To - À	CPP RPC	Pay Rémunération From - De	To - À	CPP RPC	Pay Rémunération From - De	To - À	CPP RPC
440.89 -	441.09	14.40	456.21 -	456.41	15.12	471.53 -	471.73	15.84	486.85 -	487.05	16.56
441.10 -	441.31	14.41	456.42 -	456.63	15.13	471.74 -	471.95	15.85	487.06 -	487.26	16.57
441.32 -	441.52	14.42	456.64 -	456.84	15.14	471.96 -	472.16	15.86	487.27 -	487.48	16.58
441.53 -	441.73	14.43	456.85 -	457.05	15.15	472.17 -	472.37	15.87	487.49 -	487.69	16.59
441.74 -	441.95	14.44	457.06 -	457.26	15.16	472.38 -	472.58	15.88	487.70 -	487.90	16.60
441.96 -	442.16	14.45	457.27 -	457.48	15.17	472.59 -	472.80	15.89	487.91 -	488.12	16.61
442.17 -	442.37	14.46	457.49 -	457.69	15.18	472.81 -	473.01	15.90	488.13 -	488.33	16.62
442.38 -	442.58	14.47	457.70 -	457.90	15.19	473.02 -	473.22	15.91	488.34 -	488.54	16.63
442.59 -	442.80	14.48	457.91 -	458.12	15.20	473.23 -	473.43	15.92	488.55 -	488.75	16.64
442.81 -	443.01	14.49	458.13 -	458.33	15.21	473.44 -	473.65	15.93	488.76 -	488.97	16.65
443.02 -	443.22	14.50	458.34 -	458.54	15.22	473.66 -	473.86	15.94	488.98 -	489.18	16.66
443.23 -	443.43	14.51	458.55 -	458.75	15.23	473.87 -	474.07	15.95	489.19 -	489.39	16.67
443.44 -	443.65	14.52	458.76 -	458.97	15.24	474.08 -	474.29	15.96	489.40 -	489.60	16.68
443.66 -	443.86	14.53	458.98 -	459.18	15.25	474.30 -	474.50	15.97	489.61 -	489.82	16.69
443.87 -	444.07	14.54	459.19 -	459.39	15.26	474.51 -	474.71	15.98	489.83 -	490.03	16.70
444.08 -	444.29	14.55	459.40 -	459.60	15.27	474.72 -	474.92	15.99	490.04 -	490.24	16.71
444.30 -	444.50	14.56	459.61 -	459.82	15.28	474.93 -	475.14	16.00	490.25 -	490.46	16.72
444.51 -	444.71	14.57	459.83 -	460.03	15.29	475.15 -	475.35	16.01	490.47 -	490.67	16.73
444.72 -	444.92	14.58	460.04 -	460.24	15.30	475.36 -	475.56	16.02	490.68 -	490.88	16.74
444.93 -	445.14	14.59	460.25 -	460.46	15.31	475.57 -	475.78	16.03	490.89 -	491.09	16.75
445.15 -	445.35	14.60	460.47 -	460.67	15.32	475.79 -	475.99	16.04	491.10 -	491.31	16.76
445.36 -	445.56	14.61	460.68 -	460.88	15.33	476.00 -	476.20	16.05	491.32 -	491.52	16.77
445.57 -	445.78	14.62	460.89 -	461.09	15.34	476.21 -	476.41	16.06	491.53 -	491.73	16.78
445.79 -	445.99	14.63	461.10 -	461.31	15.35	476.42 -	476.63	16.07	491.74 -	491.95	16.79
446.00 -	446.20	14.64	461.32 -	461.52	15.36	476.64 -	476.84	16.08	491.96 -	492.16	16.80
446.21 -	446.41	14.65	461.53 -	461.73	15.37	476.85 -	477.05	16.09	492.17 -	492.37	16.81
446.42 -	446.63	14.66	461.74 -	461.95	15.38	477.06 -	477.26	16.10	492.38 -	492.58	16.82
446.64 -	446.84	14.67	461.96 -	462.16	15.39	477.27 -	477.48	16.11	492.59 -	492.80	16.83
446.85 -	447.05	14.68	462.17 -	462.37	15.40	477.49 -	477.69	16.12	492.81 -	493.01	16.84
447.06 -	447.26	14.69	462.38 -	462.58	15.41	477.70 -	477.90	16.13	493.02 -	493.22	16.85
447.27 -	447.48	14.70	462.59 -	462.80	15.42	477.91 -	478.12	16.14	493.23 -	493.43	16.86
447.49 -	447.69	14.71	462.81 -	463.01	15.43	478.13 -	478.33	16.15	493.44 -	493.65	16.87
447.70 -	447.90	14.72	463.02 -	463.22	15.44	478.34 -	478.54	16.16	493.66 -	493.86	16.88
447.91 -	448.12	14.73	463.23 -	463.43	15.45	478.55 -	478.75	16.17	493.87 -	494.07	16.89
448.13 -	448.33	14.74	463.44 -	463.65	15.46	478.76 -	478.97	16.18	494.08 -	494.29	16.90
448.34 -	448.54	14.75	463.66 -	463.86	15.47	478.98 -	479.18	16.19	494.30 -	494.50	16.91
448.55 -	448.75	14.76	463.87 -	464.07	15.48	479.19 -	479.39	16.20	494.51 -	494.71	16.92
448.76 -	448.97	14.77	464.08 -	464.29	15.49	479.40 -	479.60	16.21	494.72 -	494.92	16.93
448.98 -	449.18	14.78	464.30 -	464.50	15.50	479.61 -	479.82	16.22	494.93 -	495.14	16.94
449.19 -	449.39	14.79	464.51 -	464.71	15.51	479.83 -	480.03	16.23	495.15 -	495.35	16.95
449.40 -	449.60	14.80	464.72 -	464.92	15.52	480.04 -	480.24	16.24	495.36 -	495.56	16.96
449.61 -	449.82	14.81	464.93 -	465.14	15.53	480.25 -	480.46	16.25	495.57 -	495.78	16.97
449.83 -	450.03	14.82	465.15 -	465.35	15.54	480.47 -	480.67	16.26	495.79 -	495.99	16.98
450.04 -	450.24	14.83	465.36 -	465.56	15.55	480.68 -	480.88	16.27	496.00 -	496.20	16.99
450.25 -	450.46	14.84	465.57 -	465.78	15.56	480.89 -	481.09	16.28	496.21 -	496.41	17.00
450.47 -	450.67	14.85	465.79 -	465.99	15.57	481.10 -	481.31	16.29	496.42 -	496.63	17.01
450.68 -	450.88	14.86	466.00 -	466.20	15.58	481.32 -	481.52	16.30	496.64 -	496.84	17.02
450.89 -	451.09	14.87	466.21 -	466.41	15.59	481.53 -	481.73	16.31	496.85 -	497.05	17.03
451.10 -	451.31	14.88	466.42 -	466.63	15.60	481.74 -	481.95	16.32	497.06 -	497.26	17.04
451.32 -	451.52	14.89	466.64 -	466.84	15.61	481.96 -	482.16	16.33	497.27 -	497.48	17.05
451.53 -	451.73	14.90	466.85 -	467.05	15.62	482.17 -	482.37	16.34	497.49 -	497.69	17.06
451.74 -	451.95	14.91	467.06 -	467.26	15.63	482.38 -	482.58	16.35	497.70 -	497.90	17.07
451.96 -	452.16	14.92	467.27 -	467.48	15.64	482.59 -	482.80	16.36	497.91 -	498.12	17.08
452.17 -	452.37	14.93	467.49 -	467.69	15.65	482.81 -	483.01	16.37	498.13 -	498.33	17.09
452.38 -	452.58	14.94	467.70 -	467.90	15.66	483.02 -	483.22	16.38	498.34 -	498.54	17.10
452.59 -	452.80	14.95	467.91 -	468.12	15.67	483.23 -	483.43	16.39	498.55 -	498.75	17.11
452.81 -	453.01	14.96	468.13 -	468.33	15.68	483.44 -	483.65	16.40	498.76 -	498.97	17.12
453.02 -	453.22	14.97	468.34 -	468.54	15.69	483.66 -	483.86	16.41	498.98 -	499.18	17.13
453.23 -	453.43	14.98	468.55 -	468.75	15.70	483.87 -	484.07	16.42	499.19 -	499.39	17.14
453.44 -	453.65	14.99	468.76 -	468.97	15.71	484.08 -	484.29	16.43	499.40 -	499.60	17.15
453.66 -	453.86	15.00	468.98 -	469.18	15.72	484.30 -	484.50	16.44	499.61 -	499.82	17.16
453.87 -	454.07	15.01	469.19 -	469.39	15.73	484.51 -	484.71	16.45	499.83 -	500.03	17.17
454.08 -	454.29	15.02	469.40 -	469.60	15.74	484.72 -	484.92	16.46	500.04 -	500.24	17.18
454.30 -	454.50	15.03	469.61 -	469.82	15.75	484.93 -	485.14	16.47	500.25 -	500.46	17.19
454.51 -	454.71	15.04	469.83 -	470.03	15.76	485.15 -	485.35	16.48	500.47 -	500.67	17.20
454.72 -	454.92	15.05	470.04 -	470.24	15.77	485.36 -	485.56	16.49	500.68 -	500.88	17.21
454.93 -	455.14	15.06	470.25 -	470.46	15.78	485.57 -	485.78	16.50	500.89 -	501.09	17.22
455.15 -	455.35	15.07	470.47 -	470.67	15.79	485.79 -	485.99	16.51	501.10 -	501.31	17.23
455.36 -	455.56	15.08	470.68 -	470.88	15.80	486.00 -	486.20	16.52	501.32 -	501.52	17.24
455.57 -	455.78	15.09	470.89 -	471.09	15.81	486.21 -	486.41	16.53	501.53 -	501.73	17.25
455.79 -	455.99	15.10	471.10 -	471.31	15.82	486.42 -	486.63	16.54	501.74 -	501.95	17.26
456.00 -	456.20	15.11	471.32 -	471.52	15.83	486.64 -	486.84	16.55	501.96 -	502.16	17.27

Employee's maximum CPP contribution for 2002 is $1,673.20   La cotisation maximale de l'employé au RPC pour 2002 est de 1 673,20 $ **B-19**

Canada Pension Plan Contributions
Biweekly (26 pay periods a year)

Cotisations au Régime de pensions du Canada
Aux deux semaines (26 périodes de paie par année)

Pay Rémunération From - De	To - À	CPP RPC	Pay Rémunération From - De	To - À	CPP RPC	Pay Rémunération From - De	To - À	CPP RPC	Pay Rémunération From - De	To - À	CPP RPC
1237.49	1237.69	51.84	1252.81	1253.01	52.56	1268.13	1268.33	53.28	1283.44	1283.65	54.00
1237.70	1237.90	51.85	1253.02	1253.22	52.57	1268.34	1268.54	53.29	1283.66	1283.86	54.01
1237.91	1238.12	51.86	1253.23	1253.43	52.58	1268.55	1268.75	53.30	1283.87	1284.07	54.02
1238.13	1238.33	51.87	1253.44	1253.65	52.59	1268.76	1268.97	53.31	1284.08	1284.29	54.03
1238.34	1238.54	51.88	1253.66	1253.86	52.60	1268.98	1269.18	53.32	1284.30	1284.50	54.04
1238.55	1238.75	51.89	1253.87	1254.07	52.61	1269.19	1269.39	53.33	1284.51	1284.71	54.05
1238.76	1238.97	51.90	1254.08	1254.29	52.62	1269.40	1269.60	53.34	1284.72	1284.92	54.06
1238.98	1239.18	51.91	1254.30	1254.50	52.63	1269.61	1269.82	53.35	1284.93	1285.14	54.07
1239.19	1239.39	51.92	1254.51	1254.71	52.64	1269.83	1270.03	53.36	1285.15	1285.35	54.08
1239.40	1239.60	51.93	1254.72	1254.92	52.65	1270.04	1270.24	53.37	1285.36	1285.56	54.09
1239.61	1239.82	51.94	1254.93	1255.14	52.66	1270.25	1270.46	53.38	1285.57	1285.78	54.10
1239.83	1240.03	51.95	1255.15	1255.35	52.67	1270.47	1270.67	53.39	1285.79	1285.99	54.11
1240.04	1240.24	51.96	1255.36	1255.56	52.68	1270.68	1270.88	53.40	1286.00	1286.20	54.12
1240.25	1240.46	51.97	1255.57	1255.78	52.69	1270.89	1271.09	53.41	1286.21	1286.41	54.13
1240.47	1240.67	51.98	1255.79	1255.99	52.70	1271.10	1271.31	53.42	1286.42	1286.63	54.14
1240.68	1240.88	51.99	1256.00	1256.20	52.71	1271.32	1271.52	53.43	1286.64	1286.84	54.15
1240.89	1241.09	52.00	1256.21	1256.41	52.72	1271.53	1271.73	53.44	1286.85	1287.05	54.16
1241.10	1241.31	52.01	1256.42	1256.63	52.73	1271.74	1271.95	53.45	1287.06	1287.26	54.17
1241.32	1241.52	52.02	1256.64	1256.84	52.74	1271.96	1272.16	53.46	1287.27	1287.48	54.18
1241.53	1241.73	52.03	1256.85	1257.05	52.75	1272.17	1272.37	53.47	1287.49	1287.69	54.19
1241.74	1241.95	52.04	1257.06	1257.26	52.76	1272.38	1272.58	53.48	1287.70	1287.90	54.20
1241.96	1242.16	52.05	1257.27	1257.48	52.77	1272.59	1272.80	53.49	1287.91	1288.12	54.21
1242.17	1242.37	52.06	1257.49	1257.69	52.78	1272.81	1273.01	53.50	1288.13	1288.33	54.22
1242.38	1242.58	52.07	1257.70	1257.90	52.79	1273.02	1273.22	53.51	1288.34	1288.54	54.23
1242.59	1242.80	52.08	1257.91	1258.12	52.80	1273.23	1273.43	53.52	1288.55	1288.75	54.24
1242.81	1243.01	52.09	1258.13	1258.33	52.81	1273.44	1273.65	53.53	1288.76	1288.97	54.25
1243.02	1243.22	52.10	1258.34	1258.54	52.82	1273.66	1273.86	53.54	1288.98	1289.18	54.26
1243.23	1243.43	52.11	1258.55	1258.75	52.83	1273.87	1274.07	53.55	1289.19	1289.39	54.27
1243.44	1243.65	52.12	1258.76	1258.97	52.84	1274.08	1274.29	53.56	1289.40	1289.60	54.28
1243.66	1243.86	52.13	1258.98	1259.18	52.85	1274.30	1274.50	53.57	1289.61	1289.82	54.29
1243.87	1244.07	52.14	1259.19	1259.39	52.86	1274.51	1274.71	53.58	1289.83	1290.03	54.30
1244.08	1244.29	52.15	1259.40	1259.60	52.87	1274.72	1274.92	53.59	1290.04	1290.24	54.31
1244.30	1244.50	52.16	1259.61	1259.82	52.88	1274.93	1275.14	53.60	1290.25	1290.46	54.32
1244.51	1244.71	52.17	1259.83	1260.03	52.89	1275.15	1275.35	53.61	1290.47	1290.67	54.33
1244.72	1244.92	52.18	1260.04	1260.24	52.90	1275.36	1275.56	53.62	1290.68	1290.88	54.34
1244.93	1245.14	52.19	1260.25	1260.46	52.91	1275.57	1275.78	53.63	1290.89	1291.09	54.35
1245.15	1245.35	52.20	1260.47	1260.67	52.92	1275.79	1275.99	53.64	1291.10	1291.31	54.36
1245.36	1245.56	52.21	1260.68	1260.88	52.93	1276.00	1276.20	53.65	1291.32	1291.52	54.37
1245.57	1245.78	52.22	1260.89	1261.09	52.94	1276.21	1276.41	53.66	1291.53	1291.73	54.38
1245.79	1245.99	52.23	1261.10	1261.31	52.95	1276.42	1276.63	53.67	1291.74	1291.95	54.39
1246.00	1246.20	52.24	1261.32	1261.52	52.96	1276.64	1276.84	53.68	1291.96	1292.16	54.40
1246.21	1246.41	52.25	1261.53	1261.73	52.97	1276.85	1277.05	53.69	1292.17	1292.37	54.41
1246.42	1246.63	52.26	1261.74	1261.95	52.98	1277.06	1277.26	53.70	1292.38	1292.58	54.42
1246.64	1246.84	52.27	1261.96	1262.16	52.99	1277.27	1277.48	53.71	1292.59	1292.80	54.43
1246.85	1247.05	52.28	1262.17	1262.37	53.00	1277.49	1277.69	53.72	1292.81	1293.01	54.44
1247.06	1247.26	52.29	1262.38	1262.58	53.01	1277.70	1277.90	53.73	1293.02	1293.22	54.45
1247.27	1247.48	52.30	1262.59	1262.80	53.02	1277.91	1278.12	53.74	1293.23	1293.43	54.46
1247.49	1247.69	52.31	1262.81	1263.01	53.03	1278.13	1278.33	53.75	1293.44	1293.65	54.47
1247.70	1247.90	52.32	1263.02	1263.22	53.04	1278.34	1278.54	53.76	1293.66	1293.86	54.48
1247.91	1248.12	52.33	1263.23	1263.43	53.05	1278.55	1278.75	53.77	1293.87	1294.07	54.49
1248.13	1248.33	52.34	1263.44	1263.65	53.06	1278.76	1278.97	53.78	1294.08	1294.29	54.50
1248.34	1248.54	52.35	1263.66	1263.86	53.07	1278.98	1279.18	53.79	1294.30	1294.50	54.51
1248.55	1248.75	52.36	1263.87	1264.07	53.08	1279.19	1279.39	53.80	1294.51	1294.71	54.52
1248.76	1248.97	52.37	1264.08	1264.29	53.09	1279.40	1279.60	53.81	1294.72	1294.92	54.53
1248.98	1249.18	52.38	1264.30	1264.50	53.10	1279.61	1279.82	53.82	1294.93	1295.14	54.54
1249.19	1249.39	52.39	1264.51	1264.71	53.11	1279.83	1280.03	53.83	1295.15	1295.35	54.55
1249.40	1249.60	52.40	1264.72	1264.92	53.12	1280.04	1280.24	53.84	1295.36	1295.56	54.56
1249.61	1249.82	52.41	1264.93	1265.14	53.13	1280.25	1280.46	53.85	1295.57	1295.78	54.57
1249.83	1250.03	52.42	1265.15	1265.35	53.14	1280.47	1280.67	53.86	1295.79	1295.99	54.58
1250.04	1250.24	52.43	1265.36	1265.56	53.15	1280.68	1280.88	53.87	1296.00	1296.20	54.59
1250.25	1250.46	52.44	1265.57	1265.78	53.16	1280.89	1281.09	53.88	1296.21	1296.41	54.60
1250.47	1250.67	52.45	1265.79	1265.99	53.17	1281.10	1281.31	53.89	1296.42	1296.63	54.61
1250.68	1250.88	52.46	1266.00	1266.20	53.18	1281.32	1281.52	53.90	1296.64	1296.84	54.62
1250.89	1251.09	52.47	1266.21	1266.41	53.19	1281.53	1281.73	53.91	1296.85	1297.05	54.63
1251.10	1251.31	52.48	1266.42	1266.63	53.20	1281.74	1281.95	53.92	1297.06	1297.26	54.64
1251.32	1251.52	52.49	1266.64	1266.84	53.21	1281.96	1282.16	53.93	1297.27	1297.48	54.65
1251.53	1251.73	52.50	1266.85	1267.05	53.22	1282.17	1282.37	53.94	1297.49	1297.69	54.66
1251.74	1251.95	52.51	1267.06	1267.26	53.23	1282.38	1282.58	53.95	1297.70	1297.90	54.67
1251.96	1252.16	52.52	1267.27	1267.48	53.24	1282.59	1282.80	53.96	1297.91	1298.12	54.68
1252.17	1252.37	52.53	1267.49	1267.69	53.25	1282.81	1283.01	53.97	1298.13	1298.33	54.69
1252.38	1252.58	52.54	1267.70	1267.90	53.26	1283.02	1283.22	53.98	1298.34	1298.54	54.70
1252.59	1252.80	52.55	1267.91	1268.12	53.27	1283.23	1283.43	53.99	1298.55	1298.75	54.71

B-32 Employee's maximum CPP contribution for 2002 is $1,673.20   La cotisation maximale de l'employé au RPC pour 2002 est de 1 673,20 $

Employment Insurance Premiums

Cotisations à l'assurance-emploi

Insurable Earnings Rémunération assurable		EI premium Cotisation d'AE	Insurable Earnings Rémunération assurable		EI premium Cotisation d'AE	Insurable Earnings Rémunération assurable		EI premium Cotisation d'AE	Insurable Earnings Rémunération assurable		EI premium Cotisation d'AE
From - De	To - À		From - De	To - À		From - De	To - À		From - De	To - À	
392.96	393.40	8.65	425.69	426.13	9.37	458.41	458.86	10.09	491.14	491.59	10.81
393.41	393.86	8.66	426.14	426.59	9.38	458.87	459.31	10.10	491.60	492.04	10.82
393.87	394.31	8.67	426.60	427.04	9.39	459.32	459.77	10.11	492.05	492.49	10.83
394.32	394.77	8.68	427.05	427.49	9.40	459.78	460.22	10.12	492.50	492.95	10.84
394.78	395.22	8.69	427.50	427.95	9.41	460.23	460.68	10.13	492.96	493.40	10.85
395.23	395.68	8.70	427.96	428.40	9.42	460.69	461.13	10.14	493.41	493.86	10.86
395.69	396.13	8.71	428.41	428.86	9.43	461.14	461.59	10.15	493.87	494.31	10.87
396.14	396.59	8.72	428.87	429.31	9.44	461.60	462.04	10.16	494.32	494.77	10.88
396.60	397.04	8.73	429.32	429.77	9.45	462.05	462.49	10.17	494.78	495.22	10.89
397.05	397.49	8.74	429.78	430.22	9.46	462.50	462.95	10.18	495.23	495.68	10.90
397.50	397.95	8.75	430.23	430.68	9.47	462.96	463.40	10.19	495.69	496.13	10.91
397.96	398.40	8.76	430.69	431.13	9.48	463.41	463.86	10.20	496.14	496.59	10.92
398.41	398.86	8.77	431.14	431.59	9.49	463.87	464.31	10.21	496.60	497.04	10.93
398.87	399.31	8.78	431.60	432.04	9.50	464.32	464.77	10.22	497.05	497.49	10.94
399.32	399.77	8.79	432.05	432.49	9.51	464.78	465.22	10.23	497.50	497.95	10.95
399.78	400.22	8.80	432.50	432.95	9.52	465.23	465.68	10.24	497.96	498.40	10.96
400.23	400.68	8.81	432.96	433.40	9.53	465.69	466.13	10.25	498.41	498.86	10.97
400.69	401.13	8.82	433.41	433.86	9.54	466.14	466.59	10.26	498.87	499.31	10.98
401.14	401.59	8.83	433.87	434.31	9.55	466.60	467.04	10.27	499.32	499.77	10.99
401.60	402.04	8.84	434.32	434.77	9.56	467.05	467.49	10.28	499.78	500.22	11.00
402.05	402.49	8.85	434.78	435.22	9.57	467.50	467.95	10.29	500.23	500.68	11.01
402.50	402.95	8.86	435.23	435.68	9.58	467.96	468.40	10.30	500.69	501.13	11.02
402.96	403.40	8.87	435.69	436.13	9.59	468.41	468.86	10.31	501.14	501.59	11.03
403.41	403.86	8.88	436.14	436.59	9.60	468.87	469.31	10.32	501.60	502.04	11.04
403.87	404.31	8.89	436.60	437.04	9.61	469.32	469.77	10.33	502.05	502.49	11.05
404.32	404.77	8.90	437.05	437.49	9.62	469.78	470.22	10.34	502.50	502.95	11.06
404.78	405.22	8.91	437.50	437.95	9.63	470.23	470.68	10.35	502.96	503.40	11.07
405.23	405.68	8.92	437.96	438.40	9.64	470.69	471.13	10.36	503.41	503.86	11.08
405.69	406.13	8.93	438.41	438.86	9.65	471.14	471.59	10.37	503.87	504.31	11.09
406.14	406.59	8.94	438.87	439.31	9.66	471.60	472.04	10.38	504.32	504.77	11.10
406.60	407.04	8.95	439.32	439.77	9.67	472.05	472.49	10.39	504.78	505.22	11.11
407.05	407.49	8.96	439.78	440.22	9.68	472.50	472.95	10.40	505.23	505.68	11.12
407.50	407.95	8.97	440.23	440.68	9.69	472.96	473.40	10.41	505.69	506.13	11.13
407.96	408.40	8.98	440.69	441.13	9.70	473.41	473.86	10.42	506.14	506.59	11.14
408.41	408.86	8.99	441.14	441.59	9.71	473.87	474.31	10.43	506.60	507.04	11.15
408.87	409.31	9.00	441.60	442.04	9.72	474.32	474.77	10.44	507.05	507.49	11.16
409.32	409.77	9.01	442.05	442.49	9.73	474.78	475.22	10.45	507.50	507.95	11.17
409.78	410.22	9.02	442.50	442.95	9.74	475.23	475.68	10.46	507.96	508.40	11.18
410.23	410.68	9.03	442.96	443.40	9.75	475.69	476.13	10.47	508.41	508.86	11.19
410.69	411.13	9.04	443.41	443.86	9.76	476.14	476.59	10.48	508.87	509.31	11.20
411.14	411.59	9.05	443.87	444.31	9.77	476.60	477.04	10.49	509.32	509.77	11.21
411.60	412.04	9.06	444.32	444.77	9.78	477.05	477.49	10.50	509.78	510.22	11.22
412.05	412.49	9.07	444.78	445.22	9.79	477.50	477.95	10.51	510.23	510.68	11.23
412.50	412.95	9.08	445.23	445.68	9.80	477.96	478.40	10.52	510.69	511.13	11.24
412.96	413.40	9.09	445.69	446.13	9.81	478.41	478.86	10.53	511.14	511.59	11.25
413.41	413.86	9.10	446.14	446.59	9.82	478.87	479.31	10.54	511.60	512.04	11.26
413.87	414.31	9.11	446.60	447.04	9.83	479.32	479.77	10.55	512.05	512.49	11.27
414.32	414.77	9.12	447.05	447.49	9.84	479.78	480.22	10.56	512.50	512.95	11.28
414.78	415.22	9.13	447.50	447.95	9.85	480.23	480.68	10.57	512.96	513.40	11.29
415.23	415.68	9.14	447.96	448.40	9.86	480.69	481.13	10.58	513.41	513.86	11.30
415.69	416.13	9.15	448.41	448.86	9.87	481.14	481.59	10.59	513.87	514.31	11.31
416.14	416.59	9.16	448.87	449.31	9.88	481.60	482.04	10.60	514.32	514.77	11.32
416.60	417.04	9.17	449.32	449.77	9.89	482.05	482.49	10.61	514.78	515.22	11.33
417.05	417.49	9.18	449.78	450.22	9.90	482.50	482.95	10.62	515.23	515.68	11.34
417.50	417.95	9.19	450.23	450.68	9.91	482.96	483.40	10.63	515.69	516.13	11.35
417.96	418.40	9.20	450.69	451.13	9.92	483.41	483.86	10.64	516.14	516.59	11.36
418.41	418.86	9.21	451.14	451.59	9.93	483.87	484.31	10.65	516.60	517.04	11.37
418.87	419.31	9.22	451.60	452.04	9.94	484.32	484.77	10.66	517.05	517.49	11.38
419.32	419.77	9.23	452.05	452.49	9.95	484.78	485.22	10.67	517.50	517.95	11.39
419.78	420.22	9.24	452.50	452.95	9.96	485.23	485.68	10.68	517.96	518.40	11.40
420.23	420.68	9.25	452.96	453.40	9.97	485.69	486.13	10.69	518.41	518.86	11.41
420.69	421.13	9.26	453.41	453.86	9.98	486.14	486.59	10.70	518.87	519.31	11.42
421.14	421.59	9.27	453.87	454.31	9.99	486.60	487.04	10.71	519.32	519.77	11.43
421.60	422.04	9.28	454.32	454.77	10.00	487.05	487.49	10.72	519.78	520.22	11.44
422.05	422.49	9.29	454.78	455.22	10.01	487.50	487.95	10.73	520.23	520.68	11.45
422.50	422.95	9.30	455.23	455.68	10.02	487.96	488.40	10.74	520.69	521.13	11.46
422.96	423.40	9.31	455.69	456.13	10.03	488.41	488.86	10.75	521.14	521.59	11.47
423.41	423.86	9.32	456.14	456.59	10.04	488.87	489.31	10.76	521.60	522.04	11.48
423.87	424.31	9.33	456.60	457.04	10.05	489.32	489.77	10.77	522.05	522.49	11.49
424.32	424.77	9.34	457.05	457.49	10.06	489.78	490.22	10.78	522.50	522.95	11.50
424.78	425.22	9.35	457.50	457.95	10.07	490.23	490.68	10.79	522.96	523.40	11.51
425.23	425.68	9.36	457.96	458.40	10.08	490.69	491.13	10.80	523.41	523.86	11.52

Yearly maximum insurable earnings are $39,000
Yearly maximum employee premiums are $858.00
The premium rate for 2002 is 2.20 %

Le maximum annuel de la rémunération assurable est de 39 000 $
La cotisation maximale annuelle de l'employé est de 858,00 $
La taux de cotisations pour 2002 est de 2,20 %

C-4

Employment Insurance Premiums

Cotisations à l'assurance-emploi

Insurable Earnings / Rémunération assurable		EI premium / Cotisation d'AE	Insurable Earnings / Rémunération assurable		EI premium / Cotisation d'AE	Insurable Earnings / Rémunération assurable		EI premium / Cotisation d'AE	Insurable Earnings / Rémunération assurable		EI premium / Cotisation d'AE
From - De	To - À		From - De	To - À		From - De	To - À		From - De	To - À	
1178.41 -	1178.86	25.93	1211.14 -	1211.59	26.65	1243.87 -	1244.31	27.37	1276.60 -	1277.04	28.09
1178.87 -	1179.31	25.94	1211.60 -	1212.04	26.66	1244.32 -	1244.77	27.38	1277.05 -	1277.49	28.10
1179.32 -	1179.77	25.95	1212.05 -	1212.49	26.67	1244.78 -	1245.22	27.39	1277.50 -	1277.95	28.11
1179.78 -	1180.22	25.96	1212.50 -	1212.95	26.68	1245.23 -	1245.68	27.40	1277.96 -	1278.40	28.12
1180.23 -	1180.68	25.97	1212.96 -	1213.40	26.69	1245.69 -	1246.13	27.41	1278.41 -	1278.86	28.13
1180.69 -	1181.13	25.98	1213.41 -	1213.86	26.70	1246.14 -	1246.59	27.42	1278.87 -	1279.31	28.14
1181.14 -	1181.59	25.99	1213.87 -	1214.31	26.71	1246.60 -	1247.04	27.43	1279.32 -	1279.77	28.15
1181.60 -	1182.04	26.00	1214.32 -	1214.77	26.72	1247.05 -	1247.49	27.44	1279.78 -	1280.22	28.16
1182.05 -	1182.49	26.01	1214.78 -	1215.22	26.73	1247.50 -	1247.95	27.45	1280.23 -	1280.68	28.17
1182.50 -	1182.95	26.02	1215.23 -	1215.68	26.74	1247.96 -	1248.40	27.46	1280.69 -	1281.13	28.18
1182.96 -	1183.40	26.03	1215.69 -	1216.13	26.75	1248.41 -	1248.86	27.47	1281.14 -	1281.59	28.19
1183.41 -	1183.86	26.04	1216.14 -	1216.59	26.76	1248.87 -	1249.31	27.48	1281.60 -	1282.04	28.20
1183.87 -	1184.31	26.05	1216.60 -	1217.04	26.77	1249.32 -	1249.77	27.49	1282.05 -	1282.49	28.21
1184.32 -	1184.77	26.06	1217.05 -	1217.49	26.78	1249.78 -	1250.22	27.50	1282.50 -	1282.95	28.22
1184.78 -	1185.22	26.07	1217.50 -	1217.95	26.79	1250.23 -	1250.68	27.51	1282.96 -	1283.40	28.23
1185.23 -	1185.68	26.08	1217.96 -	1218.40	26.80	1250.69 -	1251.13	27.52	1283.41 -	1283.86	28.24
1185.69 -	1186.13	26.09	1218.41 -	1218.86	26.81	1251.14 -	1251.59	27.53	1283.87 -	1284.31	28.25
1186.14 -	1186.59	26.10	1218.87 -	1219.31	26.82	1251.60 -	1252.04	27.54	1284.32 -	1284.77	28.26
1186.60 -	1187.04	26.11	1219.32 -	1219.77	26.83	1252.05 -	1252.49	27.55	1284.78 -	1285.22	28.27
1187.05 -	1187.49	26.12	1219.78 -	1220.22	26.84	1252.50 -	1252.95	27.56	1285.23 -	1285.68	28.28
1187.50 -	1187.95	26.13	1220.23 -	1220.68	26.85	1252.96 -	1253.40	27.57	1285.69 -	1286.13	28.29
1187.96 -	1188.40	26.14	1220.69 -	1221.13	26.86	1253.41 -	1253.86	27.58	1286.14 -	1286.59	28.30
1188.41 -	1188.86	26.15	1221.14 -	1221.59	26.87	1253.87 -	1254.31	27.59	1286.60 -	1287.04	28.31
1188.87 -	1189.31	26.16	1221.60 -	1222.04	26.88	1254.32 -	1254.77	27.60	1287.05 -	1287.49	28.32
1189.32 -	1189.77	26.17	1222.05 -	1222.49	26.89	1254.78 -	1255.22	27.61	1287.50 -	1287.95	28.33
1189.78 -	1190.22	26.18	1222.50 -	1222.95	26.90	1255.23 -	1255.68	27.62	1287.96 -	1288.40	28.34
1190.23 -	1190.68	26.19	1222.96 -	1223.40	26.91	1255.69 -	1256.13	27.63	1288.41 -	1288.86	28.35
1190.69 -	1191.13	26.20	1223.41 -	1223.86	26.92	1256.14 -	1256.59	27.64	1288.87 -	1289.31	28.36
1191.14 -	1191.59	26.21	1223.87 -	1224.31	26.93	1256.60 -	1257.04	27.65	1289.32 -	1289.77	28.37
1191.60 -	1192.04	26.22	1224.32 -	1224.77	26.94	1257.05 -	1257.49	27.66	1289.78 -	1290.22	28.38
1192.05 -	1192.49	26.23	1224.78 -	1225.22	26.95	1257.50 -	1257.95	27.67	1290.23 -	1290.68	28.39
1192.50 -	1192.95	26.24	1225.23 -	1225.68	26.96	1257.96 -	1258.40	27.68	1290.69 -	1291.13	28.40
1192.96 -	1193.40	26.25	1225.69 -	1226.13	26.97	1258.41 -	1258.86	27.69	1291.14 -	1291.59	28.41
1193.41 -	1193.86	26.26	1226.14 -	1226.59	26.98	1258.87 -	1259.31	27.70	1291.60 -	1292.04	28.42
1193.87 -	1194.31	26.27	1226.60 -	1227.04	26.99	1259.32 -	1259.77	27.71	1292.05 -	1292.49	28.43
1194.32 -	1194.77	26.28	1227.05 -	1227.49	27.00	1259.78 -	1260.22	27.72	1292.50 -	1292.95	28.44
1194.78 -	1195.22	26.29	1227.50 -	1227.95	27.01	1260.23 -	1260.68	27.73	1292.96 -	1293.40	28.45
1195.23 -	1195.68	26.30	1227.96 -	1228.40	27.02	1260.69 -	1261.13	27.74	1293.41 -	1293.86	28.46
1195.69 -	1196.13	26.31	1228.41 -	1228.86	27.03	1261.14 -	1261.59	27.75	1293.87 -	1294.31	28.47
1196.14 -	1196.59	26.32	1228.87 -	1229.31	27.04	1261.60 -	1262.04	27.76	1294.32 -	1294.77	28.48
1196.60 -	1197.04	26.33	1229.32 -	1229.77	27.05	1262.05 -	1262.49	27.77	1294.78 -	1295.22	28.49
1197.05 -	1197.49	26.34	1229.78 -	1230.22	27.06	1262.50 -	1262.95	27.78	1295.23 -	1295.68	28.50
1197.50 -	1197.95	26.35	1230.23 -	1230.68	27.07	1262.96 -	1263.40	27.79	1295.69 -	1296.13	28.51
1197.96 -	1198.40	26.36	1230.69 -	1231.13	27.08	1263.41 -	1263.86	27.80	1296.14 -	1296.59	28.52
1198.41 -	1198.86	26.37	1231.14 -	1231.59	27.09	1263.87 -	1264.31	27.81	1296.60 -	1297.04	28.53
1198.87 -	1199.31	26.38	1231.60 -	1232.04	27.10	1264.32 -	1264.77	27.82	1297.05 -	1297.49	28.54
1199.32 -	1199.77	26.39	1232.05 -	1232.49	27.11	1264.78 -	1265.22	27.83	1297.50 -	1297.95	28.55
1199.78 -	1200.22	26.40	1232.50 -	1232.95	27.12	1265.23 -	1265.68	27.84	1297.96 -	1298.40	28.56
1200.23 -	1200.68	26.41	1232.96 -	1233.40	27.13	1265.69 -	1266.13	27.85	1298.41 -	1298.86	28.57
1200.69 -	1201.13	26.42	1233.41 -	1233.86	27.14	1266.14 -	1266.59	27.86	1298.87 -	1299.31	28.58
1201.14 -	1201.59	26.43	1233.87 -	1234.31	27.15	1266.60 -	1267.04	27.87	1299.32 -	1299.77	28.59
1201.60 -	1202.04	26.44	1234.32 -	1234.77	27.16	1267.05 -	1267.49	27.88	1299.78 -	1300.22	28.60
1202.05 -	1202.49	26.45	1234.78 -	1235.22	27.17	1267.50 -	1267.95	27.89	1300.23 -	1300.68	28.61
1202.50 -	1202.95	26.46	1235.23 -	1235.68	27.18	1267.96 -	1268.40	27.90	1300.69 -	1301.13	28.62
1202.96 -	1203.40	26.47	1235.69 -	1236.13	27.19	1268.41 -	1268.86	27.91	1301.14 -	1301.59	28.63
1203.41 -	1203.86	26.48	1236.14 -	1236.59	27.20	1268.87 -	1269.31	27.92	1301.60 -	1302.04	28.64
1203.87 -	1204.31	26.49	1236.60 -	1237.04	27.21	1269.32 -	1269.77	27.93	1302.05 -	1302.49	28.65
1204.32 -	1204.77	26.50	1237.05 -	1237.49	27.22	1269.78 -	1270.22	27.94	1302.50 -	1302.95	28.66
1204.78 -	1205.22	26.51	1237.50 -	1237.95	27.23	1270.23 -	1270.68	27.95	1302.96 -	1303.40	28.67
1205.23 -	1205.68	26.52	1237.96 -	1238.40	27.24	1270.69 -	1271.13	27.96	1303.41 -	1303.86	28.68
1205.69 -	1206.13	26.53	1238.41 -	1238.86	27.25	1271.14 -	1271.59	27.97	1303.87 -	1304.31	28.69
1206.14 -	1206.59	26.54	1238.87 -	1239.31	27.26	1271.60 -	1272.04	27.98	1304.32 -	1304.77	28.70
1206.60 -	1207.04	26.55	1239.32 -	1239.77	27.27	1272.05 -	1272.49	27.99	1304.78 -	1305.22	28.71
1207.05 -	1207.49	26.56	1239.78 -	1240.22	27.28	1272.50 -	1272.95	28.00	1305.23 -	1305.68	28.72
1207.50 -	1207.95	26.57	1240.23 -	1240.68	27.29	1272.96 -	1273.40	28.01	1305.69 -	1306.13	28.73
1207.96 -	1208.40	26.58	1240.69 -	1241.13	27.30	1273.41 -	1273.86	28.02	1306.14 -	1306.59	28.74
1208.41 -	1208.86	26.59	1241.14 -	1241.59	27.31	1273.87 -	1274.31	28.03	1306.60 -	1307.04	28.75
1208.87 -	1209.31	26.60	1241.60 -	1242.04	27.32	1274.32 -	1274.77	28.04	1307.05 -	1307.49	28.76
1209.32 -	1209.77	26.61	1242.05 -	1242.49	27.33	1274.78 -	1275.22	28.05	1307.50 -	1307.95	28.77
1209.78 -	1210.22	26.62	1242.50 -	1242.95	27.34	1275.23 -	1275.68	28.06	1307.96 -	1308.40	28.78
1210.23 -	1210.68	26.63	1242.96 -	1243.40	27.35	1275.69 -	1276.13	28.07	1308.41 -	1308.86	28.79
1210.69 -	1211.13	26.64	1243.41 -	1243.86	27.36	1276.14 -	1276.59	28.08	1308.87 -	1309.31	28.80

Yearly maximum insurable earnings are $39,000
Yearly maximum employee premiums are $858.00
The premium rate for 2002 is 2.20 %

Le maximum annuel de la rémunération assurable est de 39 000 $
La cotisation maximale annuelle de l'employé est de 858,00 $
La taux de cotisations pour 2002 est de 2,20 %

C-10

Federal tax deductions
Effective January 1, 2002
Biweekly (26 pay periods a year)
**Also look up the tax deductions
in the provincial table**

Retenues d'impôt fédéral
En vigueur le 1er janvier 2002
Aux deux semaines (26 périodes de paie par année)
**Cherchez aussi les retenues d'impôt
dans la table provinciale**

Pay Rémunération		Federal claim codes/Codes de demande fédéraux										
		0	1	2	3	4	5	6	7	8	9	10
From De	Less than Moins de	Deduct from each pay Retenez sur chaque paie										
	310	*	.00									
310. -	314	47.50	.50									
314. -	318	48.10	1.10									
318. -	322	48.70	1.70									
322. -	326	49.30	2.30									
326. -	330	49.85	2.90									
330. -	334	50.45	3.50									
334. -	338	51.05	4.10									
338. -	342	51.65	4.70									
342. -	346	52.25	5.30	.05								
346. -	350	52.85	5.85	.65								
350. -	354	53.45	6.45	1.25								
354. -	358	54.05	7.05	1.85								
358. -	362	54.65	7.65	2.45								
362. -	366	55.25	8.25	3.05								
366. -	370	55.85	8.85	3.65								
370. -	374	56.45	9.45	4.25								
374. -	378	57.00	10.05	4.85								
378. -	382	57.60	10.65	5.45								
382. -	386	58.20	11.25	6.00								
386. -	390	58.80	11.85	6.60								
390. -	394	59.40	12.45	7.20								
394. -	398	60.00	13.00	7.80								
398. -	402	60.60	13.60	8.40								
402. -	406	61.20	14.20	9.00								
406. -	410	61.80	14.80	9.60								
410. -	414	62.40	15.40	10.20								
414. -	418	63.00	16.00	10.80	.35							
418. -	422	63.60	16.60	11.40	.95							
422. -	426	64.15	17.20	12.00	1.55							
426. -	430	64.75	17.80	12.60	2.15							
430. -	434	65.35	18.40	13.20	2.75							
434. -	438	65.95	19.00	13.75	3.35							
438. -	442	66.55	19.60	14.35	3.95							
442. -	446	67.15	20.15	14.95	4.55							
446. -	450	67.75	20.75	15.55	5.15							
450. -	454	68.35	21.35	16.15	5.75							
454. -	458	68.95	21.95	16.75	6.35							
458. -	462	69.55	22.55	17.35	6.95							
462. -	466	70.15	23.15	17.95	7.50							
466. -	470	70.70	23.75	18.55	8.10							
470. -	474	71.30	24.35	19.15	8.70							
474. -	478	71.90	24.95	19.75	9.30							
478. -	482	72.50	25.55	20.35	9.90							
482. -	486	73.10	26.15	20.90	10.50	.10						
486. -	490	73.70	26.75	21.50	11.10	.70						
490. -	494	74.30	27.30	22.10	11.70	1.30						
494. -	498	74.90	27.90	22.70	12.30	1.85						
498. -	502	75.50	28.50	23.30	12.90	2.45						
502. -	506	76.10	29.10	23.90	13.50	3.05						
506. -	510	76.70	29.70	24.50	14.10	3.65						
510. -	514	77.30	30.30	25.10	14.65	4.25						
514. -	518	77.90	30.90	25.70	15.25	4.85						
518. -	522	78.45	31.50	26.30	15.85	5.45						
522. -	526	79.05	32.10	26.90	16.45	6.05						

* You normally use claim code "0" only for non-resident employees. However, if you have non-resident employees who earn less than the minimum amount shown in the "Pay" column, you may not be able to use these tables. Instead, refer to the "Step-by-step calculation of tax deductions" in Section "A" of this publication.

* Le code de demande «0» est normalement utilisé seulement pour les non-résidents. Cependant, si la rémunération de votre employé non résidant est inférieure au montant minimum indiqué dans la colonne «Rémunération», vous ne pourrez peut-être pas utiliser ces tables. Reportez-vous alors au «Calcul des retenues d'impôt, étape par étape» dans la section «A» de cette publication.

This table is available on diskette (TOD).   D-7   **Vous pouvez obtenir cette table sur disquette (TSD).**

Federal tax deductions
Effective January 1, 2002
Biweekly (26 pay periods a year)
**Also look up the tax deductions
in the provincial table**

Retenues d'impôt fédéral
En vigueur le 1er janvier 2002
Aux deux semaines (26 périodes de paie par année)
**Cherchez aussi les retenues d'impôt
dans la table provinciale**

Pay Rémunération		Federal claim codes/Codes de demande fédéraux										
From De	Less than Moins de	0	1	2	3	4	5	6	7	8	9	10
						Deduct from each pay Retenez sur chaque paie						
966. -	982	146.10	99.10	93.90	83.50	73.05	62.65	52.25	41.80	31.40	21.00	10.55
982. -	998	148.50	101.50	96.30	85.90	75.45	65.05	54.60	44.20	33.80	23.35	12.95
998. -	1014	150.85	103.90	98.70	88.25	77.85	67.40	57.00	46.60	36.15	25.75	15.35
1014. -	1030	153.25	106.25	101.05	90.65	80.20	69.80	59.40	48.95	38.55	28.15	17.70
1030. -	1046	155.65	108.65	103.45	93.05	82.60	72.20	61.75	51.35	40.95	30.50	20.10
1046. -	1062	158.00	111.05	105.85	95.40	85.00	74.55	64.15	53.75	43.30	32.90	22.50
1062. -	1078	160.40	113.40	108.20	97.80	87.40	76.95	66.55	56.10	45.70	35.30	24.85
1078. -	1094	162.80	115.80	110.60	100.20	89.75	79.35	68.90	58.50	48.10	37.65	27.25
1094. -	1110	165.15	118.20	113.00	102.55	92.15	81.70	71.30	60.90	50.45	40.05	29.65
1110. -	1126	167.55	120.55	115.35	104.95	94.50	84.10	73.70	63.25	52.85	42.45	32.00
1126. -	1142	169.95	122.95	117.75	107.35	96.90	86.50	76.05	65.65	55.25	44.80	34.40
1142. -	1158	172.30	125.35	120.15	109.70	99.30	88.85	78.45	68.05	57.60	47.20	36.80
1158. -	1174	174.70	127.70	122.50	112.10	101.65	91.25	80.85	70.40	60.00	49.60	39.15
1174. -	1190	177.10	130.10	124.90	114.50	104.05	93.65	83.20	72.80	62.40	51.95	41.55
1190. -	1206	179.45	132.50	127.30	116.85	106.45	96.00	85.60	75.20	64.75	54.35	43.95
1206. -	1222	181.85	134.85	129.65	119.25	108.80	98.40	88.00	77.55	67.15	56.75	46.30
1222. -	1238	184.90	137.95	132.75	122.30	111.90	101.45	91.05	80.65	70.20	59.80	49.40
1238. -	1254	188.25	141.30	136.05	125.65	115.25	104.80	94.40	84.00	73.55	63.15	52.75
1254. -	1270	191.60	144.65	139.40	129.00	118.60	108.15	97.75	87.30	76.90	66.50	56.05
1270. -	1286	194.95	147.95	142.75	132.35	121.90	111.50	101.10	90.65	80.25	69.85	59.40
1286. -	1302	198.30	151.30	146.10	135.70	125.25	114.85	104.45	94.00	83.60	73.15	62.75
1302. -	1318	201.65	154.65	149.45	139.05	128.60	118.20	107.75	97.35	86.95	76.50	66.10
1318. -	1334	205.00	158.00	152.80	142.35	131.95	121.55	111.10	100.70	90.30	79.85	69.45
1334. -	1350	208.30	161.35	156.15	145.70	135.30	124.90	114.45	104.05	93.60	83.20	72.80
1350. -	1366	211.65	164.70	159.50	149.05	138.65	128.20	117.80	107.40	96.95	86.55	76.15
1366. -	1382	215.00	168.05	162.80	152.40	142.00	131.55	121.15	110.75	100.30	89.90	79.45
1382. -	1398	218.35	171.35	166.15	155.75	145.35	134.90	124.50	114.05	103.65	93.25	82.80
1398. -	1414	221.70	174.70	169.50	159.10	148.65	138.25	127.85	117.40	107.00	96.60	86.15
1414. -	1430	225.05	178.05	172.85	162.45	152.00	141.60	131.20	120.75	110.35	99.90	89.50
1430. -	1446	228.40	181.40	176.20	165.75	155.35	144.95	134.50	124.10	113.70	103.25	92.85
1446. -	1462	231.70	184.75	179.55	169.10	158.70	148.30	137.85	127.45	117.05	106.60	96.20
1462. -	1478	235.05	188.10	182.90	172.45	162.05	151.65	141.20	130.80	120.35	109.95	99.55
1478. -	1494	238.40	191.45	186.20	175.80	165.40	154.95	144.55	134.15	123.70	113.30	102.90
1494. -	1510	241.75	194.80	189.55	179.15	168.75	158.30	147.90	137.50	127.05	116.65	106.25
1510. -	1526	245.25	198.30	193.10	182.65	172.25	161.80	151.40	141.00	130.55	120.15	109.75
1526. -	1542	248.80	201.80	196.60	186.20	175.75	165.35	154.95	144.50	134.10	123.65	113.25
1542. -	1558	252.30	205.35	200.10	189.70	179.30	168.85	158.45	148.05	137.60	127.20	116.75
1558. -	1574	255.85	208.85	203.65	193.20	182.80	172.40	161.95	151.55	141.15	130.70	120.30
1574. -	1590	259.35	212.35	207.15	196.75	186.30	175.90	165.50	155.05	144.65	134.25	123.80
1590. -	1606	262.85	215.90	210.70	200.25	189.85	179.40	169.00	158.60	148.15	137.75	127.35
1606. -	1622	266.40	219.40	214.20	203.80	193.35	182.95	172.55	162.10	151.70	141.25	130.85
1622. -	1638	269.90	222.95	217.70	207.30	196.90	186.45	176.05	165.65	155.20	144.80	134.35
1638. -	1654	273.45	226.45	221.25	210.80	200.40	190.00	179.55	169.15	158.75	148.30	137.90
1654. -	1670	276.95	229.95	224.75	214.35	203.90	193.50	183.10	172.65	162.25	151.85	141.40
1670. -	1686	280.45	233.50	228.30	217.85	207.45	197.00	186.60	176.20	165.75	155.35	144.95
1686. -	1702	284.00	237.00	231.80	221.40	210.95	200.55	190.15	179.70	169.30	158.85	148.45
1702. -	1718	287.50	240.55	235.30	224.90	214.50	204.05	193.65	183.25	172.80	162.40	151.95
1718. -	1734	291.05	244.05	238.85	228.40	218.00	207.60	197.15	186.75	176.35	165.90	155.50
1734. -	1750	294.55	247.55	242.35	231.95	221.50	211.10	200.70	190.25	179.85	169.45	159.00
1750. -	1766	298.05	251.10	245.90	235.45	225.05	214.60	204.20	193.80	183.35	172.95	162.55
1766. -	1782	301.60	254.60	249.40	239.00	228.55	218.15	207.75	197.30	186.90	176.45	166.05
1782. -	1798	305.10	258.15	252.90	242.50	232.10	221.65	211.25	200.85	190.40	180.00	169.55
1798. -	1814	308.65	261.65	256.45	246.00	235.60	225.20	214.75	204.35	193.95	183.50	173.10
1814. -	1830	312.15	265.15	259.95	249.55	239.10	228.70	218.30	207.85	197.45	187.05	176.60
1830. -	1846	315.65	268.70	263.50	253.05	242.65	232.20	221.80	211.40	200.95	190.55	180.15

This table is available on diskette (TOD).　　　　D-9　　　　Vous pouvez obtenir cette table sur disquette (TSD).

Ontario

Provincial tax deductions effective January 1, 2002
Biweekly (26 pay periods a year)
**Also look up the tax deductions
in the federal table**

Ontario
Retenues d'impôt provincial en vigueur le 1er janvier 2002
Aux deux semaines (26 périodes de paie par année)
**Cherchez aussi les retenues d'impôt
dans la table fédérale**

Pay Rémunération		Provincial claim codes/Codes de demande provinciaux										
From De	Less than Moins de	0	1	2	3	4	5	6	7	8	9	10
		Deduct from each pay Retenez sur chaque paie										
	422	*	.00									
422. -	426	24.25	.40									
426. -	430	24.50	.85									
430. -	434	24.70	1.30									
434. -	438	24.95	1.75									
438. -	442	25.15	2.20									
442. -	446	25.40	2.65									
446. -	450	25.60	3.10									
450. -	454	25.85	3.55									
454. -	458	26.05	4.00	.15								
458. -	462	26.30	4.45	.60								
462. -	466	26.50	4.90	1.05								
466. -	470	26.75	5.35	1.50								
470. -	474	26.95	5.80	1.95								
474. -	478	27.20	6.25	2.40								
478. -	482	27.40	6.70	2.85								
482. -	486	27.65	7.15	3.30								
486. -	490	27.85	7.60	3.75								
490. -	494	28.10	8.05	4.20								
494. -	498	28.30	8.50	4.65								
498. -	502	28.55	8.95	5.10								
502. -	506	28.75	9.40	5.55								
506. -	510	29.00	9.85	6.00								
510. -	514	29.20	10.30	6.45								
514. -	518	29.45	10.75	6.90								
518. -	522	29.65	11.20	7.35								
522. -	526	29.90	11.65	7.80	.10							
526. -	530	30.10	12.10	8.25	.55							
530. -	534	30.35	12.45	8.70	1.00							
534. -	538	30.55	12.70	9.15	1.45							
538. -	542	30.80	12.90	9.60	1.90							
542. -	546	31.00	13.15	10.05	2.35							
546. -	550	31.25	13.35	10.50	2.80							
550. -	554	31.45	13.60	10.95	3.25							
554. -	558	31.70	13.80	11.40	3.70							
558. -	562	31.95	14.05	11.85	4.15							
562. -	566	32.15	14.25	12.30	4.60							
566. -	570	32.40	14.50	12.55	5.05							
570. -	574	32.60	14.70	12.80	5.50							
574. -	578	32.85	14.95	13.00	5.95							
578. -	582	33.05	15.15	13.25	6.40							
582. -	586	33.30	15.40	13.45	6.85							
586. -	590	33.50	15.60	13.70	7.30							
590. -	594	33.75	15.85	13.90	7.75	.05						
594. -	598	33.95	16.05	14.15	8.20	.50						
598. -	602	34.20	16.30	14.35	8.65	.95						
602. -	606	34.40	16.50	14.60	9.10	1.40						
606. -	610	34.65	16.75	14.80	9.55	1.85						
610. -	614	34.85	16.95	15.05	10.00	2.30						
614. -	618	35.10	17.20	15.25	10.45	2.75						
618. -	622	35.30	17.40	15.50	10.90	3.20						
622. -	626	35.55	17.65	15.70	11.35	3.65						
626. -	630	35.75	17.85	15.95	11.80	4.10						
630. -	634	36.00	18.10	16.15	12.25	4.55						
634. -	638	36.20	18.30	16.40	12.55	5.00						

* You normally use claim code "0" only for non-resident employees. However, if you have non-resident employees who earn less than the minimum amount shown in the "Pay" column, you may not be able to use these tables. Instead, refer to the "Step-by-step calculation of tax deductions" in Section "A" of this publication.

* Le code de demande «0» est normalement utilisé seulement pour les non-résidents. Cependant, si la rémunération de votre employé non résidant est inférieure au montant minimum indiqué dans la colonne «Rémunération», vous ne pourrez peut-être pas utiliser ces tables. Reportez-vous alors au «Calcul des retenues d'impôt, étape par étape» dans la section «A» de cette publication.

This table is available on diskette (TOD).   E-7   Vous pouvez obtenir cette table sur disquette (TSD).

Provincial tax deductions effective January 1, 2002
Biweekly (26 pay periods a year)
**Also look up the tax deductions
in the federal table**

Retenues d'impôt provincial en vigueur le 1er janvier 2002
Aux deux semaines (26 périodes de paie par année)
**Cherchez aussi les retenues d'impôt
dans la table fédérale**

Pay			Provincial claim codes/Codes de demande provinciaux										
Rémunération			0	1	2	3	4	5	6	7	8	9	10
From De	Less than Moins de						Deduct from each pay Retenez sur chaque paie						
1078.	-	1094	61.55	43.65	41.75	37.90	34.05	30.20	26.35	22.45	18.60	14.75	9.45
1094.	-	1110	62.45	44.55	42.65	38.80	34.95	31.10	27.25	23.40	19.50	15.65	11.25
1110.	-	1126	63.35	45.45	43.55	39.70	35.85	32.00	28.15	24.30	20.40	16.55	12.70
1126.	-	1142	64.25	46.35	44.45	40.60	36.75	32.90	29.05	25.20	21.30	17.45	13.60
1142.	-	1158	65.15	47.25	45.35	41.50	37.65	33.80	29.95	26.10	22.25	18.35	14.50
1158.	-	1174	66.05	48.15	46.25	42.40	38.55	34.70	30.85	27.00	23.15	19.25	15.40
1174.	-	1190	66.95	49.05	47.15	43.30	39.45	35.60	31.75	27.90	24.05	20.15	16.30
1190.	-	1206	67.85	50.00	48.05	44.20	40.35	36.50	32.65	28.80	24.95	21.10	17.20
1206.	-	1222	68.75	50.90	48.95	45.10	41.25	37.40	33.55	29.70	25.85	22.00	18.10
1222.	-	1238	69.75	51.85	49.95	46.10	42.25	38.40	34.55	30.70	26.80	22.95	19.10
1238.	-	1254	71.15	53.25	51.35	47.50	43.65	39.80	35.95	32.05	28.20	24.35	20.50
1254.	-	1270	72.55	54.65	52.75	48.90	45.05	41.20	37.30	33.45	29.60	25.75	21.90
1270.	-	1286	73.95	56.05	54.15	50.30	46.45	42.55	38.70	34.85	31.00	27.15	23.30
1286.	-	1302	75.35	57.45	55.55	51.70	47.85	43.95	40.10	36.25	32.40	28.55	24.70
1302.	-	1318	76.75	58.85	56.95	53.10	49.20	45.35	41.50	37.65	33.80	29.95	26.10
1318.	-	1334	78.15	60.25	58.35	54.45	50.60	46.75	42.90	39.05	35.20	31.35	27.50
1334.	-	1350	79.55	61.65	59.70	55.85	52.00	48.15	44.30	40.45	36.60	32.75	28.90
1350.	-	1366	80.95	63.05	61.10	57.25	53.40	49.55	45.70	41.85	38.00	34.15	30.30
1366.	-	1382	82.35	64.45	62.50	58.65	54.80	50.95	47.10	43.25	39.40	35.55	31.70
1382.	-	1398	83.75	65.85	63.90	60.05	56.20	52.35	48.50	44.65	40.80	36.95	33.10
1398.	-	1414	85.10	67.25	65.30	61.45	57.60	53.75	49.90	46.05	42.20	38.35	34.50
1414.	-	1430	86.50	68.65	66.70	62.85	59.00	55.15	51.30	47.45	43.60	39.75	35.90
1430.	-	1446	87.90	70.05	68.10	64.25	60.40	56.55	52.70	48.85	45.00	41.15	37.30
1446.	-	1462	89.30	71.45	69.50	65.65	61.80	57.95	54.10	50.25	46.40	42.55	38.70
1462.	-	1478	90.70	72.85	70.90	67.05	63.20	59.35	55.50	51.65	47.80	43.95	40.05
1478.	-	1494	92.10	74.20	72.30	68.45	64.60	60.75	56.90	53.05	49.20	45.30	41.45
1494.	-	1510	93.50	75.60	73.70	69.85	66.00	62.15	58.30	54.45	50.60	46.70	42.85
1510.	-	1526	94.95	77.10	75.15	71.30	67.45	63.60	59.75	55.90	52.05	48.20	44.35
1526.	-	1542	96.45	78.55	76.60	72.75	68.90	65.05	61.20	57.35	53.50	49.65	45.80
1542.	-	1558	97.90	80.00	78.10	74.25	70.40	66.50	62.65	58.80	54.95	51.10	47.25
1558.	-	1574	99.35	81.50	79.55	75.70	71.85	68.00	64.15	60.30	56.45	52.60	48.70
1574.	-	1590	100.80	82.95	81.00	77.15	73.30	69.45	65.60	61.75	57.90	54.05	50.20
1590.	-	1606	102.30	84.40	82.50	78.60	74.75	70.90	67.05	63.20	59.35	55.50	51.65
1606.	-	1622	103.75	85.85	83.95	80.10	76.25	72.40	68.55	64.65	60.80	56.95	53.10
1622.	-	1638	105.20	87.35	85.40	81.55	77.70	73.85	70.00	66.15	62.30	58.45	54.60
1638.	-	1654	106.70	88.80	86.85	83.00	79.15	75.30	71.45	67.60	63.75	59.90	56.05
1654.	-	1670	108.15	90.25	88.35	84.50	80.65	76.75	72.90	69.05	65.20	61.35	57.50
1670.	-	1686	109.60	91.70	89.80	85.95	82.10	78.25	74.40	70.55	66.70	62.80	58.95
1686.	-	1702	111.05	93.20	91.25	87.40	83.55	79.70	75.85	72.00	68.15	64.30	60.45
1702.	-	1718	112.55	94.65	92.70	88.85	85.00	81.15	77.30	73.45	69.60	65.75	61.90
1718.	-	1734	114.00	96.10	94.20	90.35	86.50	82.65	78.80	74.90	71.05	67.20	63.35
1734.	-	1750	115.45	97.60	95.65	91.80	87.95	84.10	80.25	76.40	72.55	68.70	64.85
1750.	-	1766	116.95	99.05	97.10	93.25	89.40	85.55	81.70	77.85	74.00	70.15	66.30
1766.	-	1782	118.40	100.50	98.60	94.75	90.85	87.00	83.15	79.30	75.45	71.60	67.75
1782.	-	1798	119.85	101.95	100.05	96.20	92.35	88.50	84.65	80.80	76.90	73.05	69.20
1798.	-	1814	121.30	103.45	101.50	97.65	93.80	89.95	86.10	82.25	78.40	74.55	70.70
1814.	-	1830	122.80	104.90	102.95	99.10	95.25	91.40	87.55	83.70	79.85	76.00	72.15
1830.	-	1846	124.25	106.35	104.45	100.60	96.75	92.90	89.00	85.15	81.30	77.45	73.60
1846.	-	1862	125.70	107.85	105.90	102.05	98.20	94.35	90.50	86.65	82.80	78.95	75.05
1862.	-	1878	127.20	109.30	107.35	103.50	99.65	95.80	91.95	88.10	84.25	80.40	76.55
1878.	-	1894	128.65	110.75	108.85	105.00	101.10	97.25	93.40	89.55	85.70	81.85	78.00
1894.	-	1910	130.10	112.20	110.30	106.45	102.60	98.75	94.90	91.05	87.15	83.30	79.45
1910.	-	1926	131.55	113.70	111.75	107.90	104.05	100.20	96.35	92.50	88.65	84.80	80.95
1926.	-	1942	133.05	115.15	113.20	109.35	105.50	101.65	97.80	93.95	90.10	86.25	82.40
1942.	-	1958	134.50	116.60	114.70	110.85	107.00	103.10	99.25	95.40	91.55	87.70	83.85

This table is available on diskette (TOD).   E-9   Vous pouvez obtenir cette table sur disquette (TSD).

Cash Disbursements

Date	Particulars	Cheque Number	Amount Paid Out	Office Rent Maintenance	Office Supplies	Medical Supplies	Telephone	Heat and Hydro	Wages
Column Totals									

191

DATE _____

TO _____

FOR _____

Bank of Dalriada
BD
Caledonia Square
345 Bruce Road
Toronto, ON F2X 4G8

Previous Balance	$
Cheque Amount	$
Balance Forward	$

192

DATE _____

TO _____

FOR _____

Bank of Dalriada
BD
Caledonia Square
345 Bruce Road
Toronto, ON F2X 4G8

Previous Balance	$
Cheque Amount	$
Balance Forward	$

191

ARGYLL CLINIC
2999 RENFIELD STREET
TORONTO, ON F2L 4X6

DATE _____

PAY TO THE
ORDER OF _____ $ _____

_____ /100 DOLLARS

Bank of Dalriada
BD
Caledonia Square
345 Bruce Road
Toronto, ON F2X 4G8

MEMO _____

"001111" :001100 000

This form is for instructional use

192

ARGYLL CLINIC
2999 RENFIELD STREET
TORONTO, ON F2L 4X6

DATE _____

PAY TO THE
ORDER OF _____ $ _____

_____ /100 DOLLARS

Bank of Dalriada
BD
Caledonia Square
345 Bruce Road
Toronto, ON F2X 4G8

MEMO _____

"001111" :001100 000

This form is for instructional use

Stub 193 (top right)

DATE _____

TO _____

FOR _____

Bank of Dalriada

BD

Caledonia Square
345 Bruce Road
Toronto, ON F2X 4G8

Previous Balance	$
Cheque Amount	$
Balance Forward	$

193

Stub 194 (middle left)

DATE _____

TO _____

FOR _____

Bank of Dalriada

BD

Caledonia Square
345 Bruce Road
Toronto, ON F2X 4G8

Previous Balance	$
Cheque Amount	$
Balance Forward	$

194

Cheque 193 (bottom right)

ARGYLL CLINIC
2999 RENFIELD STREET
TORONTO, ON F2L 4X6

DATE _____

PAY TO THE
ORDER OF _____

$ _____

/100 DOLLARS

Bank of Dalriada

BD

Caledonia Square
345 Bruce Road
Toronto, ON F2X 4G8

MEMO _____

This form is for
instructional use

"001111" :001100   000

193

Cheque 194 (bottom left)

ARGYLL CLINIC
2999 RENFIELD STREET
TORONTO, ON F2L 4X6

DATE _____

PAY TO THE
ORDER OF _____

$ _____

/100 DOLLARS

Bank of Dalriada

BD

Caledonia Square
345 Bruce Road
Toronto, ON F2X 4G8

MEMO _____

This form is for
instructional use

"001111" :001100   000

194

FORM D

"AS IS" LICENSE AGREEMENT AND LIMITED WARRANTY

READ THIS LICENSE CAREFULLY BEFORE USING THIS PACKAGE. BY USING THIS PACKAGE, YOU ARE AGREEING TO THE TERMS AND CONDITIONS OF THIS LICENSE. IF YOU DO NOT AGREE, DO NOT OPEN THE PACKAGE. PROMPTLY RETURN THE UNOPENED PACKAGE AND ALL ACCOMPANYING ITEMS TO THE PLACE YOU OBTAINED THEM. THESE TERMS APPLY TO ALL LICENSED SOFTWARE ON THE DISK EXCEPT THAT THE TERMS FOR USE OF ANY SHAREWARE OR FREEWARE ON THE DISKETTES ARE AS SET FORTH IN THE ELECTRONIC LICENSE LOCATED ON THE DISK:

1. GRANT OF LICENSE and OWNERSHIP: The enclosed computer programs <<and any data>> ("Software") are licensed, not sold, to you by Pearson Education Canada Inc. ("We" or the "Company") in consideration of your adoption of the accompanying Company textbooks and/or other materials, and your agreement to these terms. You own only the disk(s) but we and/or our licensors own the Software itself. This license allows instructors and students enrolled in the course using the Company textbook that accompanies this Software (the "Course") to use and display the enclosed copy of the Software for academic use only, so long as you comply with the terms of this Agreement. You may make one copy for back up only. We reserve any rights not granted to you.

2. USE RESTRICTIONS: You may not sell or license copies of the Software or the Documentation to others. You may not transfer, distribute or make available the Software or the Documentation, except to instructors and students in your school who are users of the adopted Company textbook that accompanies this Software in connection with the course for which the textbook was adopted. You may not reverse engineer, disassemble, decompile, modify, adapt, translate or create derivative works based on the Software or the Documentation. You may be held legally responsible for any copying or copyright infringement which is caused by your failure to abide by the terms of these restrictions.

3. TERMINATION: This license is effective until terminated. This license will terminate automatically without notice from the Company if you fail to comply with any provisions or limitations of this license. Upon termination, you shall destroy the Documentation and all copies of the Software. All provisions of this Agreement as to limitation and disclaimer of warranties, limitation of liability, remedies or damages, and our ownership rights shall survive termination.

4. DISCLAIMER OF WARRANTY: THE COMPANY AND ITS LICENSORS MAKE NO WARRANTIES ABOUT THE SOFTWARE, WHICH IS PROVIDED "AS-IS." IF THE DISK IS DEFECTIVE IN MATERIALS OR WORKMANSHIP, YOUR ONLY REMEDY IS TO RETURN IT TO THE COMPANY WITHIN 30 DAYS FOR REPLACEMENT UNLESS THE COMPANY DETERMINES IN GOOD FAITH THAT THE DISK HAS BEEN MISUSED OR IMPROPERLY INSTALLED, REPAIRED, ALTERED OR DAMAGED. THE COMPANY DISCLAIMS ALL WARRANTIES, EXPRESS OR IMPLIED, INCLUDING WITHOUT LIMITATION, THE IMPLIED WARRANTIES OF MERCHANTABILITY AND FITNESS FOR A PARTICULAR PURPOSE. THE COMPANY DOES NOT WARRANT, GUARANTEE OR MAKE ANY REPRESENTATION REGARDING THE ACCURACY, RELIABILITY, CURRENTNESS, USE, OR RESULTS OF USE, OF THE SOFTWARE.

5. LIMITATION OF REMEDIES AND DAMAGES: IN NO EVENT, SHALL THE COMPANY OR ITS EMPLOYEES, AGENTS, LICENSORS OR CONTRACTORS BE LIABLE FOR ANY INCIDENTAL, INDIRECT, SPECIAL OR CONSEQUENTIAL DAMAGES ARISING OUT OF OR IN CONNECTION WITH THIS LICENSE OR THE SOFTWARE, INCLUDING, WITHOUT LIMITATION, LOSS OF USE, LOSS OF DATA, LOSS OF INCOME OR PROFIT, OR OTHER LOSSES SUSTAINED AS A RESULT OF INJURY TO ANY PERSON, OR LOSS OF OR DAMAGE TO PROPERTY, OR CLAIMS OF THIRD PARTIES, EVEN IF THE COMPANY OR AN AUTHORIZED REPRESENTATIVE OF THE COMPANY HAS BEEN ADVISED OF THE POSSIBILITY OF SUCH DAMAGES. SOME JURISDICTIONS DO NOT ALLOW THE LIMITATION OF DAMAGES IN CERTAIN CIRCUMSTANCES, SO THE ABOVE LIMITATIONS MAY NOT ALWAYS APPLY.

6. GENERAL: THIS AGREEMENT SHALL BE CONSTRUED AND INTERPRETED ACCORDING TO THE LAWS OF THE PROVINCE OF ONTARIO. This Agreement is the complete and exclusive statement of the agreement between you and the Company and supersedes all proposals, prior agreements, oral or written, and any other communications between you and the company or any of its representatives relating to the subject matter.

Should you have any questions concerning this agreement or if you wish to contact the Company for any reason, please contact in writing: Customer Service, Pearson Education Canada, 26 Prince Andrew Place, Don Mills, Ontario M3C 2T8.